PRAISE FOR THE TOOTH BIBLE

As a parent of two children, ages 8 and 14, the world of pediatric dental care and orthodontics has been a "learn on and as needed basis" for many of us. This book is packed with useful, easy-to-digest information that will undoubtedly help any parent understand oral health and preventative care as their child develops. As a sleep specialist, dental health is a much misunderstood and overlooked area in sleep and breathing, and this book will be a useful tool for parents who are struggling in this arena and unsure of next steps.

-Shelby Harris, PsyD, DBSM
Clinical associate professor, Departments of Neurology and Psychiatry,
Albert Einstein College of Medicine, NYC, NY

Among the many books on the market about pregnancy and baby's health, there's a noticeable void in educating parents about their children's dental journey. This book effectively fills that gap with clear language and illustrative pictures, often answering questions I hadn't yet considered. It has eased my anxiety about dental health and enabled me to have more productive discussions with our pediatric dentist. I know I'll continue to return to The Tooth Bible as my children grow older and new questions arise. Highly recommend!

-Emily Goldberg MS, CGC
Licensed, Certified Genetic Counselor

This book is an invaluable resource for parents seeking to understand their child's dental development. As an orthodontist and mother of two, I often share this book with my patients and friends. The book demystifies the often complex world of orthodontics with clarity and precision, making it accessible and engaging. From explaining the importance of early orthodontic evaluations to detailing the phases of treatment, Dr. Geiman provides practical advice and expert insights that are both enlightening and reassuring. This book is a must-read for any parent looking to ensure their child's healthy and beautiful smile.

-Anu Nellissery DMD, MS
Orthodontist, Windsor, CT

As a pediatric dentist, I see countless children for their first ever dental visit. Unfortunately, I am often diagnosing early childhood cavities and significant bite issues. Many of these problems could be avoided if parents knew how to steer clear of certain mistakes. There is a clear lack of emphasis on oral healthcare and proper dental hygiene for newborns and toddlers. Thankfully, The Tooth Bible has stepped in to fill that void with a concise and easy to read book. It is a must-have for every family's bookshelf.

-David Berkower DDS
Pediatric Dentist, New York City, NY

The Tooth Bible by Robert Geiman and Michael Sultan is an easy to read and thorough guide. I have 3 children all going through different developmental milestones. It can be hard to stay up to speed on each of their needs. This book allows me to get the answers I am looking for in one spot. It is a reference I use for my children but also can relate to my own adult dental health. The Q&A style makes this book easy to pick up when a question arises with answers that I can understand without a dental background. As a visual learner the pictures along the way are a great aide. The Tooth Bible is a perfect title because it will serve as our family's dental reference!

-Jennie Allegretta
Interior Designer, Trietta Interiors

Prior to the arrival of my daughter, I read lots about developmental milestones and activities to ensure her health and happiness. However, when her first tooth came in, my wife and I did not know if we should brush it and we certainly did not know when we should take her to her first dental visit. The Tooth Bible efficiently outlines what every parent must know about their child's dental development. I plan to keep this book handy and reference it frequently as my daughter grows and hits new dental and developmental milestones.

-Major Paul Pikman, DO
Pulmonologist, Boston, MA

THE TOOTH BIBLE

A Parent's Guide to their Child's Smile

ROBERT GEIMAN DDS MA MS
and MICHAEL SULTAN DDS

The Tooth Bible™
© 2024 The Tooth Bible LLC,

All rights reserved. No part of this publication may be reproduced, distributed, or transmitted in any form or by any means, including photocopying, recording, or other electronic or mechanical methods, without the prior written permission of the publisher, except in the case of brief quotations embodied in critical reviews and certain other noncommercial uses permitted by copyright law.

ISBN 979-8-35094-180-7
eBook ISBN 979-8-35094-181-4

To Ian, Leora and Tanya: Your smiles are my daily inspiration. Thank you.
-RG

To my family…thank you for all that you do.
- MS

ABOUT THE AUTHORS

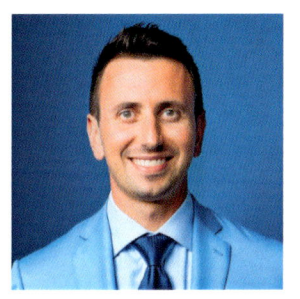

Dr. Robert "Bobby" Geiman, a Diplomate of the American Board of Orthodontics, is full-time in private practice on the Connecticut shoreline. He is also an attending at Yale New Haven Hospital, where he teaches residents on a variety of topics, including facial growth and development, orthodontic diagnosis, and orthodontic treatment planning. Dr. Geiman received his dental training at Columbia University where he completed a dual degree program: Doctor of Dental Surgery (DDS) and MA (Master of Arts in Dental Education). He went on to further his education at the University of Maryland's orthodontic program. When he's not doing something related to teeth, you can catch him playing tennis, skiing, bird watching, or spending time with his family.

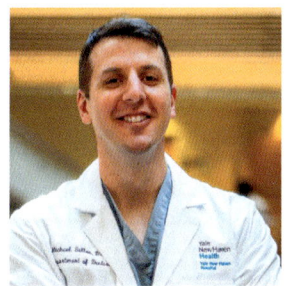

Dr. Michael Sultan is a board-certified pediatric dentist who received his Doctor of Dental Surgery from New York University: College of Dentistry, graduating with honors and induction in Omicron Kappa Upsilon, the National Dental Honor Society. He completed his post-graduate training in the specialty of Pediatric Dentistry at Yale New Haven Hospital. Dr. Sultan has published research articles in both domestic and international dental journals. He currently serves as Program Director for Yale New Haven Hospital's Pediatric Dental Residency program where he oversees the care of thousands of children annually while simultaneously training the next generation of pediatric dentists.

ADDITIONAL CONTRIBUTORS

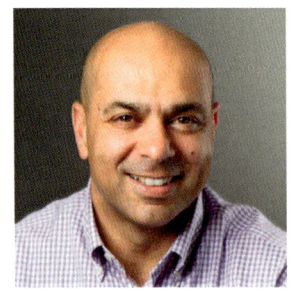

David Karas, MD is a pediatric otolaryngologist (ENT) with over twenty years of experience serving patients on the Connecticut shoreline. Dr. Karas specializes in the medical and surgical treatment of disorders of the ear, nose, throat, head, and neck in pediatric patients. He has published numerous articles and book chapters and has lectured nationally and internationally. He was the chief of Pediatric Otolaryngology at Yale New Haven Hospital and Yale Medical School for over twenty years.

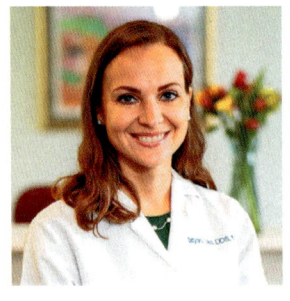

Tatyana Oks, DDS, MS, a Diplomate of the American Board of Periodontology, is a partner at River Valley Periodontics and Implant Dentistry, a private practice in southeastern Connecticut. Dr. Oks received her Doctor of Dental Surgery degree from Columbia University College of Dental Medicine and went on to earn her Master of Science degree in Periodontics from the same prestigious institution. Following graduation, Dr. Oks served on Dean's Faculty at the University of Maryland School of Dentistry, where she taught clinical periodontics. Dr. Oks is an active member of the local dental community and most recently served as president of the Shoreline Dental Society. With extensive education and clinical expertise, Dr. Oks is committed to providing exceptional periodontal care to her patients.

CONTENTS

Chapter 1 - The Importance of a Smile 5

Chapter 2 - In Utero and Birth 9

Chapter 3 - Age Zero to Three – Tiny Tooth Tales 14

Chapter 4 - Age Three to Six – Molar Milestones 32

Chapter 5 - Ages Six to Eight – Tooth Fairy Fables 48

Chapter 6 - Age Eight to Ten – An Incisor Intermission 71

Chapter 7 - Age Ten to Twelve – Tween Tooth Tell-Alls 81

Chapter 8 - Age Twelve and Beyond – Permanent Perfection 91

Chapter 9 - Orthodontics 104

Chapter 10 - Genetics 142

Chapter 11 - Gum Health 150

Chapter 12 - Airway and Sleep 160

Conclusion 165

The Tooth Bible's Smile Shop with our Recommended Product List 166

DISCLAIMER

The contents and recommendations in this book are based solely on the opinions and conclusions of the authors drawn from their clinical experience. It is crucial that the reader understand that any advice provided is not meant to be, nor can be, considered a replacement for consulting with the appropriate healthcare professional, especially in matters related to dental health.

Recommendations and examples of procedures, treatments, and results, may differ from a reader's individual experience. Readers are advised to exercise their own judgement and seek professional advice as needed, and assume all risks for using the contents of this book in lieu of consultation with the appropriate healthcare professional.

The authors do not assume any liability for the advice and recommendations provided herein. This book is intended to serve as a general guide and an educational and informational resource only. This book does not establish a doctor-patient relationship. The authors and associated individuals explicitly disclaim any responsibility for any adverse effects or consequences resulting from the use of the information presented.

The inclusion of patient photos has been done with the explicit consent from the patient and/or their parent(s).

PREFACE

After years of meeting families through dental school, residency, and then my private practice, it became apparent to me that most parents are not very knowledgeable about their children's teeth. Why would they be? It's not a topic that is taught anywhere and many parents simply don't know where to look for trustworthy answers. As if parenting isn't hard enough, most moms and dads don't have the time to focus on teeth. Some even skip their own dental appointments. Parents have a myriad of other responsibilities that seem to get a higher priority. But your child's teeth are important, and they need some attention too!

When new patients come into my office for their first appointment, I hear a few statements repeatedly: *I wish I'd known some of this stuff earlier! I feel guilty. Should I have noticed this on my own? Where can I find more information like this so I know what to look for in my other kids?* It is these questions and the sentiments behind them that inspired me to write this book. I wanted to create an easy-to-read, quick Q&A style guide that would allow parents to become more knowledgeable about and comfortable with their children's dental health. You will notice that the chapters of this book are separated by either age or topic to allow for easy reference. So sit back and relax, let's embark on this educational journey together. You are going to see and learn a lot of important information about your child's teeth, and even your own!

-Robert Geiman

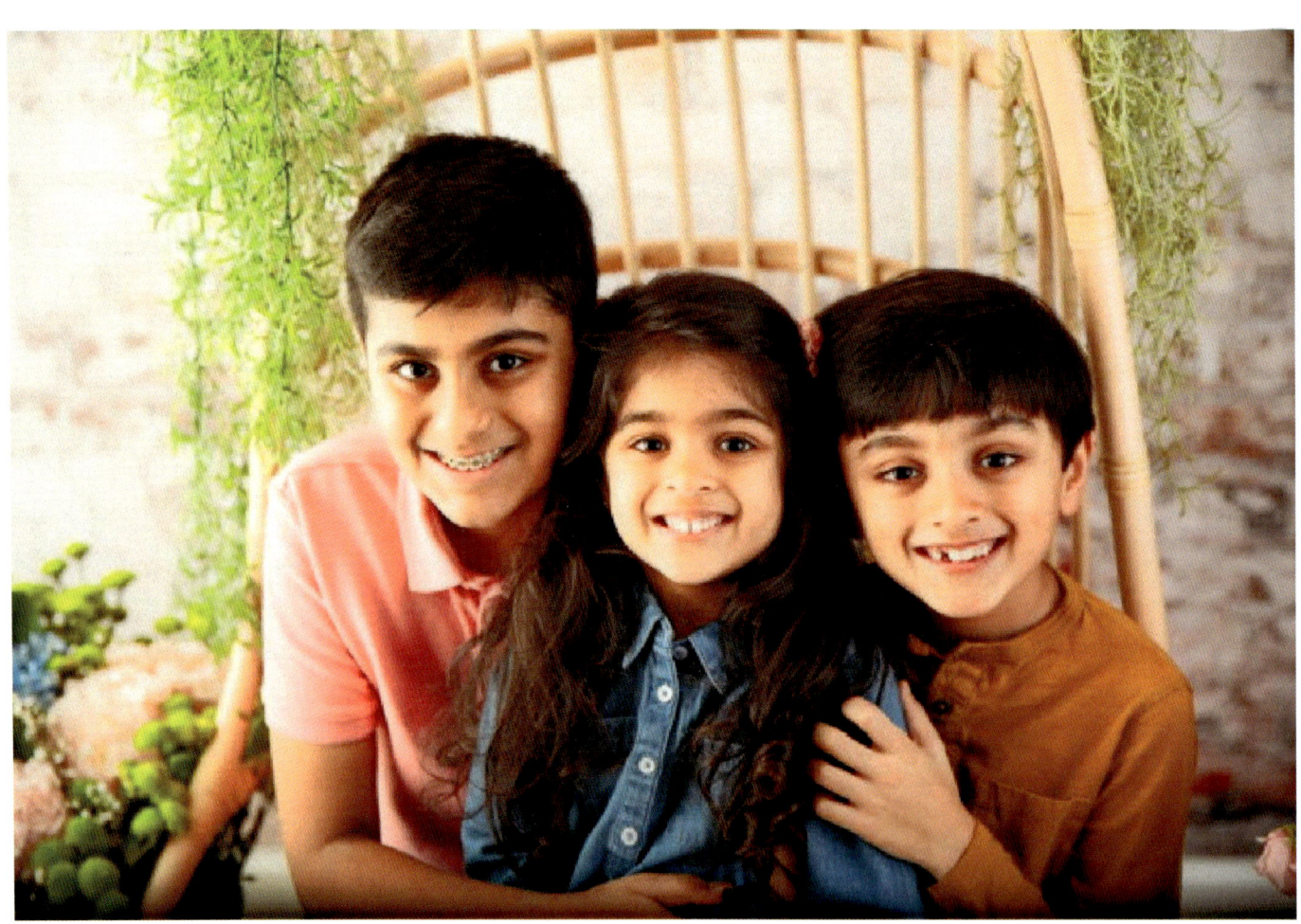

CHAPTER 1
THE IMPORTANCE OF A SMILE

First impressions are everything. As human beings, we are quick to pass judgment on others, and form opinions so strong that they can supersede even the truth itself. For better or worse, our society is one that values physical appearances in this decision making process, and it is no secret that our smiles are a crucial component to the way we present ourselves to the world. When making a first impression, a warm radiant smile may be more impactful than any words we could ever say. People associate smiles with confidence, attractiveness, approachability, and worth—desirable traits for friends, employers, and romantic partners alike. Yet for many, their smiles are a source of internal dissatisfaction. "I always used to hide my smile because I was so ashamed of my teeth," is a phrase heard far too often from patients. One can only wonder how the trajectory of their lives would have been altered if only they had the confidence to smile. Imagine what doors could have opened to them if they had the willingness and means to make a change.

As our world becomes more and more digital, the importance of image and a beautiful smile has never been more essential. A strong handshake doesn't go far on a video call...but your smile does. Despite our reservations, children today are growing up in a constant "selfie" mode where their online persona can mean as much to them as their real world presence. Giving them a smile that they are proud of, one that they aren't afraid to put on full display, might be among the most important things you can ever do for them and their self-esteem.

Why is a healthy smile important?

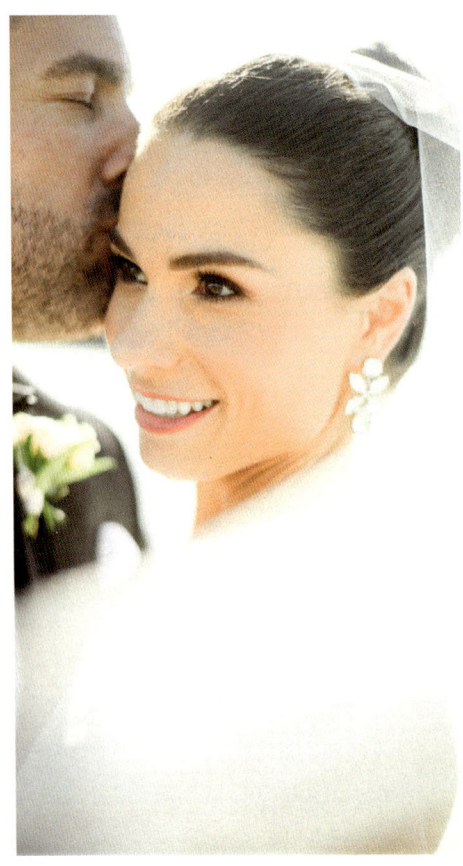

Speaking, singing, chewing, showing emotion, and bestowing beauty...the list goes on and on. With so much at stake, it is essential we keep our smiles healthy; and having a healthy smile starts with having healthy teeth. Historically, the teeth have been thought of as "separate" or "distinct" from the rest of the body. They have their own doctors, insurance plans, and even their own aisle in convenience stores. Yet, nothing could be further from the truth. The teeth are just as connected to the body as the heart, lungs and brain. People with healthy teeth tend to have an improved immune system, lower blood sugar, reduced blood pressure, as well as less stress. There are even studies linking the frequency and intensity of smiling to a longer lifespan and improved quality of life. Conversely, poor oral health leads to cavities, gum disease, bite issues, and tooth loss. These conditions have been associated with heart disease, stroke, diabetes, rheumatoid arthritis, chronic inflammation, and pregnancy-related issues. Clearly the impact our oral health has on our overall well-being is tremendous—both positive and negative.

What role does oral health play in digestion?

Digestion is the process of breaking down food into nutrients our body can absorb. The teeth kick-start this chain of events by mechanically breaking down large portions of food into smaller pieces more suitable to swallow. Humans have different types of teeth that work together to accomplish this goal. *Incisors* are the front teeth used for cutting and biting into food. *Canines* are at the corners of the mouth and are used for ripping and tearing food apart. *Molars* are in the back, and primarily chew and grind the food down. While the teeth mechanically process the food, saliva works hand-in-hand to chemically degrade and lubricate the pieces to allow for swallowing. Humans require a healthy diet of carbohydrates, proteins and lipids.

Those who have lost their teeth often must rely on softer, more processed foods, which are usually not as nutritious and healthy. A poor diet can have a host of negative consequences on your child's overall health.

What role does oral health play in speech?

Try saying the letter "F" without using your teeth to contact your lower lip. Unless you're a ventriloquist... we bet you can't do it. Now try an "S," "V," or "Z" without the use of your front teeth. The point is that the relative positions of the tongue, lips, and teeth profoundly influence our ability to produce the desired sounds. We must have both the appropriate anatomy and ability to move our oral structures in order to generate proper speech. In an unhealthy state, children or adults may develop a lisp or similar speech impairment. The capacity to communicate is essential for a developing child, with deficits putting them at risk for social and academic delay.

What role does oral health play in esthetics?

Beyond the beauty we attribute to a healthy smile, the teeth also play a significant role in giving structure to the face. Their presence is essential to provide both length and fullness. Consider how the face appears in a newborn or an elderly person in the absence of teeth; the dimensions appear short and collapsed. With tooth loss also comes a narrowing of the face, causing the cheeks to look sunken. While these problems are most often found in older individuals, they can happen in children too. Always remember that the patterns of behavior established in a child's formative years lead to the clinical picture we see in adulthood.

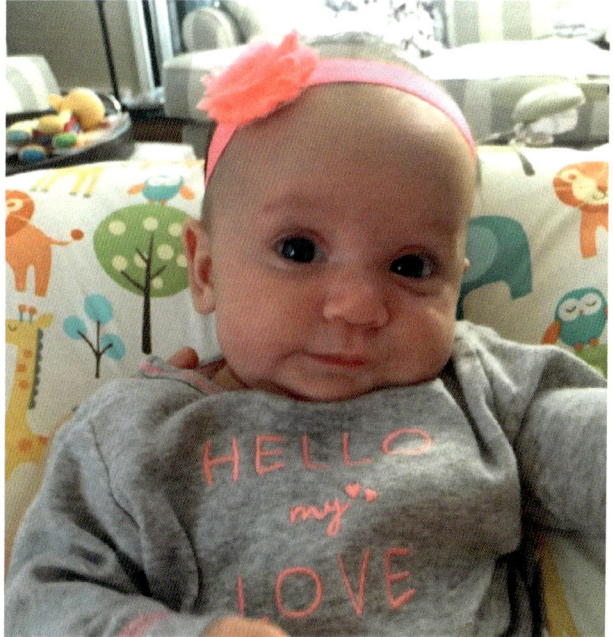

A four-month-old baby with no teeth, leading to a small lower third of the face.

Why do we have different sets of teeth?

Humans have two sets of teeth that come into the mouth during their lifetime. Each set of teeth is known as a *dentition*. The first set of *primary teeth* (or "baby teeth") will eventually be replaced by a second set made up of *permanent teeth* (or "adult teeth"). As we mature, our bodies continue to change, growing in size until we reach adulthood. The individual parts of our body generally follow suit; for example, our arms, legs, and torso lengthen as we age. Our teeth are an exception to this rule. Once a tooth is fully formed, it can no longer change proportions along with our growing body. Instead, our small baby teeth are replaced with a larger set of adult teeth that are better suited to the functional needs of the body as an adult.

"A smile is the light in the window of the soul indicating that the heart is at home."

-Christian D. Larson

A smile is so much more than a collection of teeth. It tells a tale about our lives. Next time you see someone's smile, think about the story it can tell you. Does it speak to a lifetime of meticulous love and care? Or is it a tragedy of neglect and unfortunate circumstance? As a parent, you will have the opportunity and privilege to author part of your child's "smile story"—it's a big responsibility and one you shouldn't take for granted. We hope this brief introduction has convinced you of the many reasons why a smile is worth protecting, and now that you know the *why*, it's time to delve into the *how*.

CHAPTER 2
IN UTERO AND BIRTH

Congratulations on your journey to parenthood! Whether you're planning to become pregnant, already expecting, or just welcoming your new little one, it's important to understand the impact that the in utero and birth experience can have on your child's developing mouth. Believe it or not, the formation of one's smile starts before life even begins. Our bodies have the blueprint stored in our DNA and construction commences while we are still in our mother's womb. As we make our way through life, the early choices that affect our smiles will reverberate through time.

When do baby teeth begin to form?

The development of the primary teeth ("baby teeth") begins at six weeks in the womb.[1] This initial growth occurs at the cellular level beneath the gums. First, the pattern of the tooth's size and shape is laid out, and later a hardening process known as *calcification* occurs. The earliest signs of this calcification, when minerals are added to harden the teeth, can be observed around fourteen weeks in utero.[2]

How long does it take for a tooth to fully form?

The formation process of a tooth, from the start of calcification to its ultimate completion can range from several years for baby teeth, to approximately a decade and a half for adult teeth. Even though the tooth may look fully formed when it first comes into the mouth, the tooth's root, which is the portion of the tooth under the gums, is still developing.

Can anything affect my child's teeth while I'm pregnant?

Absolutely! Your child's life is intricately tied to your own at this stage. Any insult to your body can affect your developing baby. This is the reason one should avoid smoking and drinking alcohol during pregnancy. This is also the reason why understanding the timeline for tooth development is so important. A mature tooth is strong, but an immature tooth, one that has not yet fully calcified, is fragile and susceptible to damage. Since all the baby teeth are still developing in the womb, they are all at risk when exposed to significant insults and foreign agents. Common maternal stressors that can impact the developing teeth include bacterial or viral infections during pregnancy, the use of antibiotics, high-grade fevers, and vitamin deficiencies. Depending on the magnitude and duration of the disruption, the teeth may become discolored, misshapen, or softer than normal.

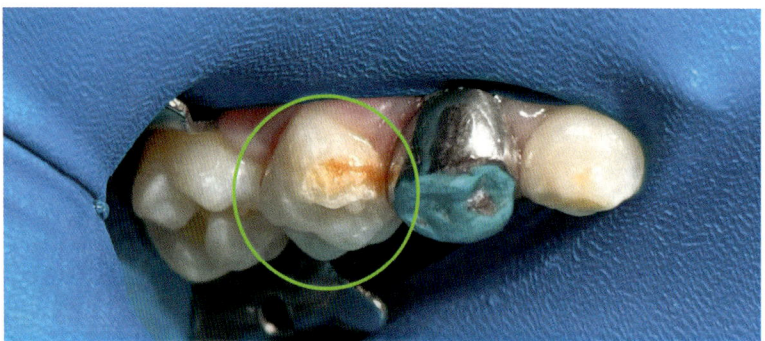

Localized area of enamel disruption seen on an upper primary molar.

How does labor and delivery affect the teeth?

The birth of a baby is a momentous and stressful occasion for both mother and child. As your baby transitions from the womb to the world, there is a dramatic change in their environment. Where the umbilical cord once provided everything your baby needed, they must now become reliant on their own body to survive. This monumental shift affects the cells that are building the teeth. If you were to look at a tooth under a microscope, you would be able to see a clear structural change corresponding to when this birth event occurred.

I've heard that babies can be born with teeth. Is that possible?

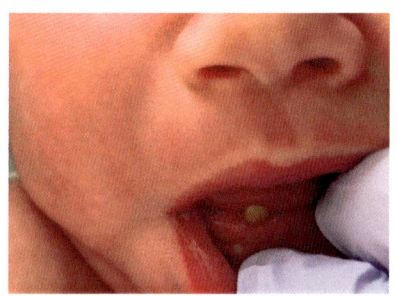

Newborn with a natal tooth in the lower incisor region.

Have you ever had a party guest show up three-hours before the time on the invite? Well…it can happen with teeth too. A tooth present at birth is known as a *natal tooth*. If the tooth emerges within the first month of life, it is known as a *neonatal tooth*. It's an uncommon occurrence, but most of the time these "early bird" teeth do not signify anything beyond premature development. However, in some rarer cases, a natal tooth can be an indicator of an underlying medical syndrome.

Is it safe to get dental care while pregnant?

Yes, it is safe! You should not neglect your own dental care during pregnancy. In fact, improving your oral health care while pregnant can reduce the risk of complications of dental diseases to both the mother and developing child.[3] While it may be reasonable to defer certain elective procedures until after delivery, the key takeaway is that *necessary* dental care can be delivered safely during any trimester. Just ensure your dentist is aware of your pregnancy so that they can take the appropriate precautions during your visit.

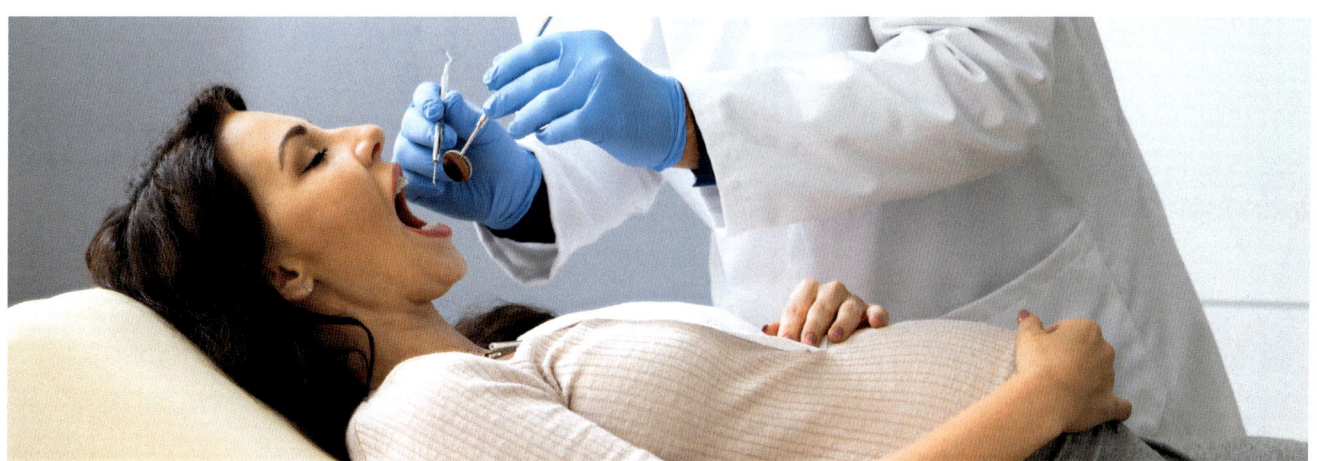

Does periodontal disease during pregnancy affect my developing child?

Periodontal disease, which will be discussed in greater detail in Chapter 11, is a bacterial infection that leads to inflammation and destruction of the supporting structures of our teeth. Some studies have shown that mothers with periodontal disease are more prone to giving birth prematurely or having low birth-weight babies.[4,5] The risk may be as much as four times greater to experience these negative birth outcomes in the presence of unhealthy gums.[6] Knowing this, if you or your partner are considering starting a family, make sure to prioritize your own oral health!

What is cleft lip or cleft lip and palate (CLP)? When, how, and why does it occur?

A *cleft* is a rare but important finding that can have profound lasting effects on your child. The issue begins between the sixth and tenth week in utero when two portions of the lip and/or the palate (roof of the mouth) do not fully connect, leaving a gap between these oral structures. This defect can cause difficulties with speech, feeding, hearing, and socialization. CLP affects one in seven hundred births and is most prevalent in Asian populations, and least common in African populations. In 70 percent of cases, the cleft is an isolated finding, and not associated with any other medical issues or syndromes.[7]

If your child is born with a cleft lip, cleft palate, or both, they will require specialized care throughout childhood and into early adulthood. CLP teams, composed of dentists, orthodontists, oral surgeons, speech pathologists, and social workers, can be found in major hospitals. The American Cleft Palate-Craniofacial Association provides a search tool, accessible by typing "ACPA Find a Team" into your search engine, which can locate the closest team based on your address and desired driving radius.

"Plan for what is difficult while it is easy, do what is great while it is small."

– Sun Tzu

The birth of your child will herald joyous new beginnings and a whirlwind of changes. Your pregnancy is a great time to start preparing for what is to come. Do not allow your child's oral health to become a distant afterthought in the face of the mounting demands of parenthood. Ready yourself with knowledge, plan for the future, and you will be well-equipped to meet the challenges ahead.

CHAPTER 3
AGE ZERO TO THREE – TINY TOOTH TALES

Babies begin their lives completely reliant on their caregivers for survival. Every feeding, every bath, every trip to the pediatrician is an exercise in dependence. But, within a year, they'll be cruising and crawling, and some may even start walking to explore the world around them. While you learn the ropes of parenthood, your baby is learning right alongside you. Their brain nearly doubles in size during this first year of life. Somehow, through all the stroller rides, sleepless nights, and the occasional diaper blowout, your infant becomes a toddler. Soon they are getting into anything and everything around your home. They'll be eating so much food that you'll wonder where they're putting it all! It's such an exciting time for both child and parent...and guess what? Your child's smile is developing hand-in-hand every step of the way.

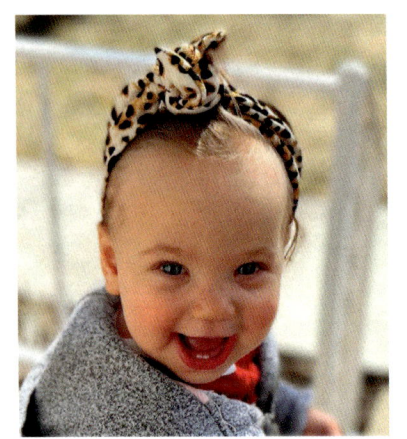

A baby who recently got her first two teeth in.

When will my child's teeth start coming in?

The first baby teeth that typically emerge are the two bottom front ones, called the lower central incisors. The process of a tooth breaking through the gums and coming into the mouth is known as *eruption*. On average, these teeth will erupt at about seven-months of age.

What teeth come next?

Next in line are usually the top two front teeth. These upper central incisors are generally larger and more square-shaped compared to their lower counterparts. They usually join the party at six- to ten-months.

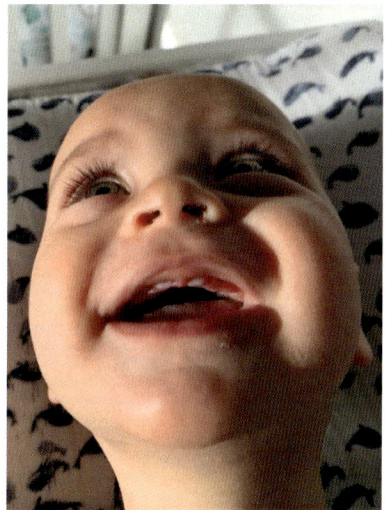 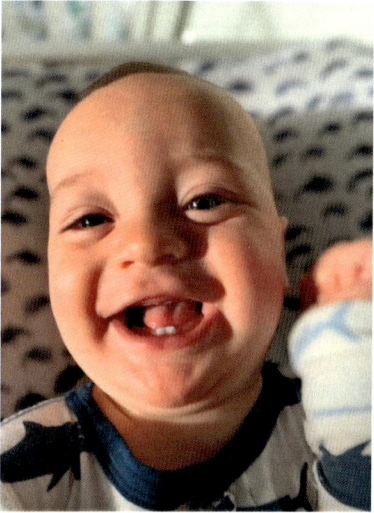

A ten-month-old starting to get their upper incisors.

What is teething? And how do I deal with it?

As a tooth forces its way through the gums, it is normal for your child to exhibit signs of discomfort, such as irritability, crankiness, biting and chewing on objects, or excessive drooling. It's also possible for the child's temperature to rise, but usually not enough to consider the child feverish (100.4°F or greater).

The good news is not all children get teething pain, but for those that do, there are various remedies you can try at home to alleviate their discomfort. Try rubbing your child's gums with a clean finger or wet gauze to provide pressure and relieve pain. Having the child bite on chilled objects, such as teething rings, typically helps as well. When children are inconsolable, over-the-counter pain relievers like ibuprofen (Advil) or acetaminophen (Tylenol) may also be used. We recommend against the use of topical anesthetics containing the active ingredient benzocaine in this age group, as well as avoiding homeopathic medications that haven't been evaluated for safety and efficacy by the Food and Drug Administration (FDA).

Does teething cause ear infections?

It's unlikely. While there may seem to be a correlation between the two based on timing, many children experience ear infections in the absence of teething, while others still experience teething with no signs of ear infection. Little children may be unable to express the source of their discomfort, and so they may often rub or tug at their ears in response to teething pain. Infections are ultimately caused by bacteria and viruses, not teething itself.

At what age should a child first visit the dentist?

According to the American Academy of Pediatric Dentistry, the recommended time for a child's first dental visit is either six-months after the eruption of their first tooth, or at one year of age, whichever occurs first.[8]

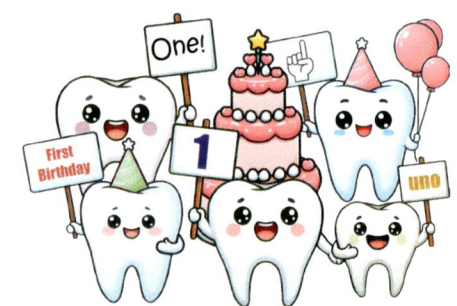

My child barely has any teeth. Why bother going so early?

This early visit allows the dentist not only a chance to examine the child for any current problems and abnormalities, but also gives them the opportunity to provide *anticipatory guidance*.

What is anticipatory guidance?

Anticipatory guidance is a term used to describe the proactive counseling that dentists provide to parents about their children's oral health. The earlier you and your child's dental education begins, the better long-term outcomes you can expect. You will learn answers to questions you never knew you had, and your family will become more familiar with the setting and members of the dental team. Your goal is to establish a *dental home*, a relationship that can provide continuous, quality, family-centered care for your child. So please don't hesitate…reap the rewards of early intervention!

Does my child need to see a pediatric dentist? Or can I take them to my general dentist?

While all dentists can choose to treat kids, pediatric dentists have completed an additional two- to three-year residency program focused solely on the dental health of children. Pediatric dentists may be better equipped to provide guidance to parents, manage uncooperative children, treat dental injuries, and provide specialized services like sedation. Children with disabilities may also highly benefit from being seen by pediatric dentists who are often more familiar with rarer conditions and their dental implications. That being said, there are many family dentists who provide excellent care to children of all ages. Talk to your dentist regarding their comfort level and experience with children prior to making a decision on where to establish care.

Some dentists have a DDS after their name but others have a DMD. What's the difference?

Sorry to diminish any folklore, but there is actually no substantive difference between the two degrees. Both the Doctor of Dental Surgery (DDS) and Doctor of Medical Dentistry (DMD) have the same academic requirements. The distinction between the two degrees is simply a matter of tradition, with some schools conferring one and some conferring the other.

Is there a predictable pattern to the rest of the teeth coming in?

After the front teeth (central incisors) have emerged, we can reasonably expect a new quartet of teeth to erupt every four-months or so until the entire set of baby teeth is complete. The pattern typically proceeds from the front of the mouth to the back, with the exception of the canines that are initially skipped over for the first set of molars. Another common trend is for the lower teeth to erupt slightly before their upper counterparts. Refer to the eruption chart on the following page for specific times.

What if my child's teeth aren't coming in on schedule?

Remain calm! There is great variability as to when teeth erupt, as illustrated by the ranges in time on the associated eruption chart. Just because your child's teeth may be delayed, doesn't necessarily indicate a problem; they may just be a "late bloomer" when it comes to dental development. However, in some situations when the timing or order of eruption is *significantly* irregular, it could indicate an underlying issue. Some things to consider when teeth do not erupt on or close to schedule include a missing tooth, pathology blocking eruption, or a lack of signaling for eruption. If your child has yet to get any baby teeth in by age one, it is recommended to consult a dentist. Lucky for you, you've already learned to see a dentist by age one anyway!

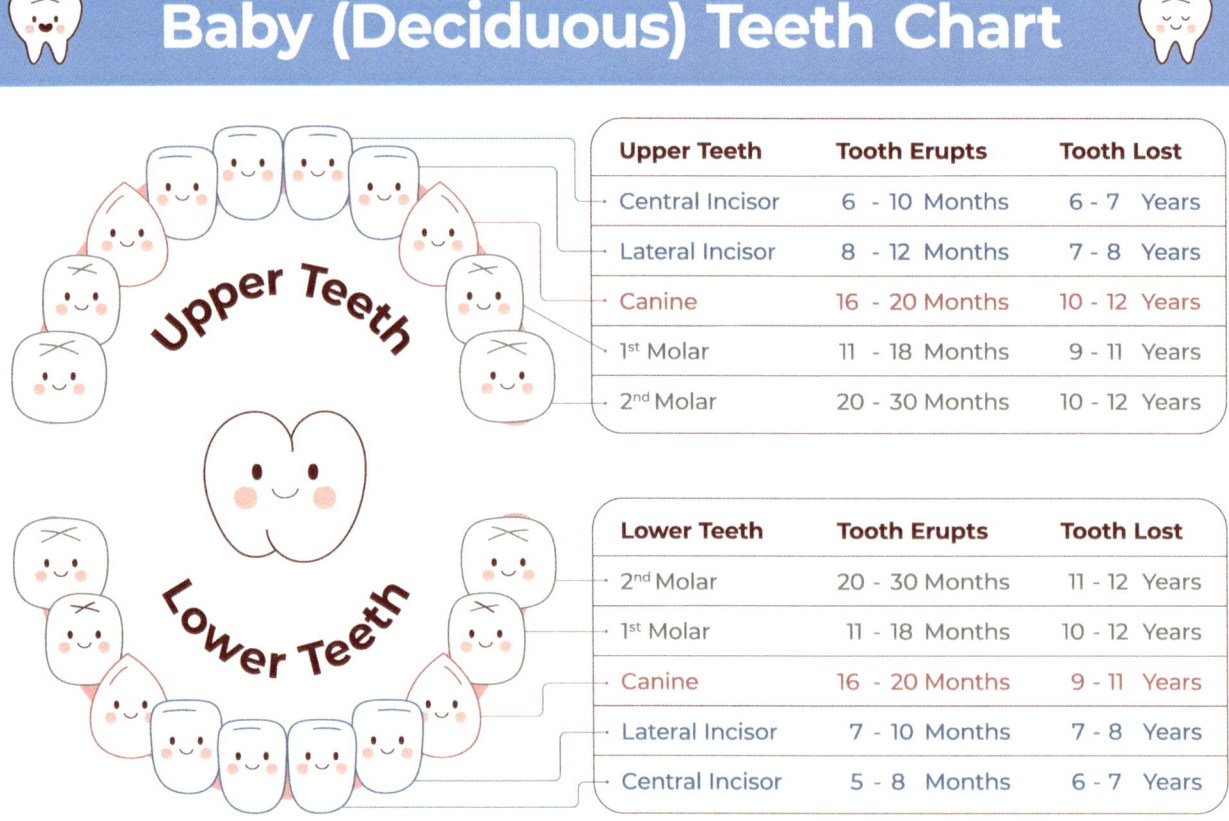

Baby (Deciduous) Teeth Chart

Upper Teeth	Tooth Erupts	Tooth Lost
Central Incisor	6 - 10 Months	6 - 7 Years
Lateral Incisor	8 - 12 Months	7 - 8 Years
Canine	16 - 20 Months	10 - 12 Years
1st Molar	11 - 18 Months	9 - 11 Years
2nd Molar	20 - 30 Months	10 - 12 Years

Lower Teeth	Tooth Erupts	Tooth Lost
2nd Molar	20 - 30 Months	11 - 12 Years
1st Molar	11 - 18 Months	10 - 12 Years
Canine	16 - 20 Months	9 - 11 Years
Lateral Incisor	7 - 10 Months	7 - 8 Years
Central Incisor	5 - 8 Months	6 - 7 Years

When should all the primary teeth (baby teeth) be in the mouth?

The typical age for a child to have all twenty of their primary teeth is around three years old. There should be ten on top and a matching ten on the bottom. Dentists (in the United States) name baby teeth with letters—from tooth #A to #T, while adult teeth are denoted by numbers starting from #1 and ending with #32.

My child has a blue/purple bump on their gums. Should I be concerned?

A bump like this is usually not a cause for concern. This swelling is most likely an *eruption hematoma*, also known as an *eruption cyst*. It is a small, fluid-filled cyst that surrounds an erupting tooth while it is emerging through the gums. The cyst may appear black, blue, or purple and is most often found associated with the erupting incisors or molars. Most of the time, these fluid-filled sacs will rupture on their own without any intervention. Once the tooth inside the cyst breaks through the gums, the pressure is released and the fluid drains away. If the discolored area has not resolved within a few weeks however, please have it evaluated by a dentist.

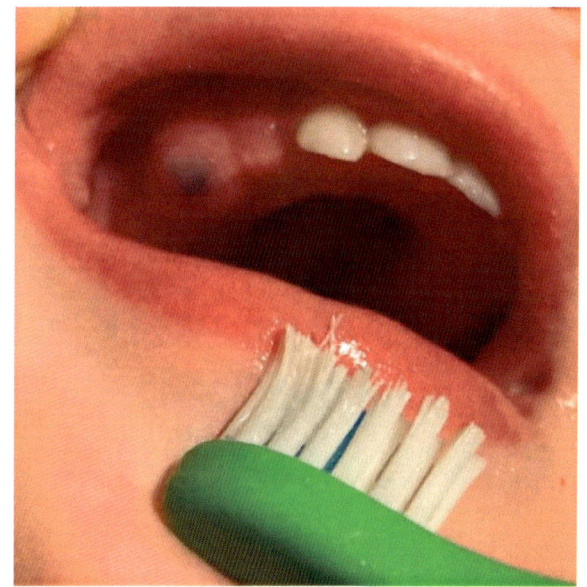

Eruption Cyst

When should I start brushing my child's teeth?

This question is of paramount importance! Simply put, as soon as teeth are in the mouth, they should be brushed. This is because as soon as teeth are in the mouth, they are susceptible to getting *cavities*.

What is a cavity?

Our bodies, including our mouths, are home to many different species of *bacteria*—some good, some bad. Among the bad bacteria are a number of species that make homes for themselves on our teeth. These bacteria use sugars derived from the carbohydrates in our diet as their source of food and energy. When these bacteria feast on sugar, they produce acid as a byproduct. Given enough time, these acids cause our teeth to break down. If the hard outer shell of a tooth, known as the *enamel*, is broken, you get what is essentially a hole in the tooth—a cavity. Dentists will sometimes refer to this process of tooth decomposition as *decay*. Small cavities are often difficult to see with the naked eye, which is why dentists will use special instruments and X-rays to check for decay. An important concept to understand is that cavities cannot fix themselves and will only get worse with time. When decay goes unnoticed or untreated, it grows and spreads.

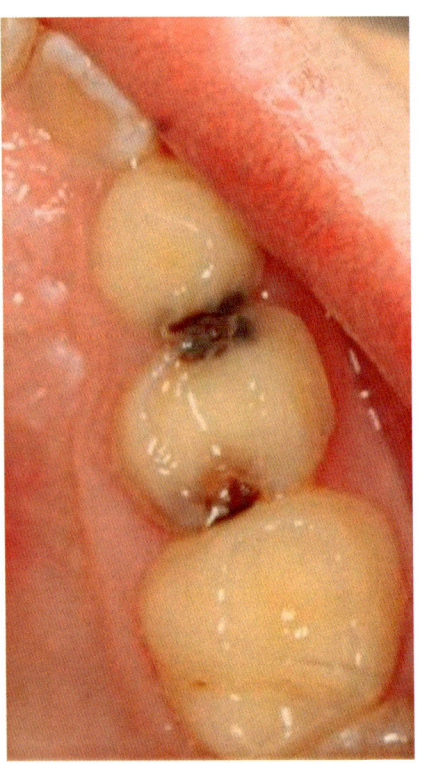

Cavities seen on a primary molar. The dark regions on the sides of the tooth are cavities.

Where do the bacteria that cause cavities come from?

Most studies on the matter suggest that mothers are typically the source of their children's cavity-causing bacteria.[9] These bacteria are often transferred from a mother's mouth to her child's through *saliva-sharing activities*. You can reduce the risk of this transmission by avoiding behaviors that introduce your own saliva into your child's mouth. These include pre-tasting or pre-chewing a child's food, sharing utensils, or placing a pacifier or bottle nipple in a child's mouth after it has been in their mother's. Mothers can also reduce the risk of transmission by taking care of their own oral health. By addressing a mother's cavities, a dentist can help reduce the total number of bacteria that can then be spread to their child.[10] It's a "two birds with one stone" scenario—by fixing your own cavities you can simultaneously help yourself and your child!

How should I brush my child's teeth at this age?

Parents should brush their children's teeth using a small soft-bristled brush twice daily. The ideal times for brushing are once in the morning, and again at night before bedtime. It is most important to ensure that brushing is done after the last meal (or drink) of the day. Employ a gentle back-and-forth scrubbing motion to remove any debris from the tooth surface. Some children at this age will not mind having their teeth brushed, but many will resist and cry. While this may sometimes be a struggle, the consequences of not brushing far outweigh the temporary challenge.

My child resists brushing. Are there any tips for controlling their head or hands?

You can gently restrain a small child by standing behind them and reaching around one of their shoulders to brush. This position may decrease unwanted movements and improve parental control. An extra set of hands can also be useful if the child is really giving you trouble. Try recruiting a spouse or older sibling to help aid in the process. If still unsuccessful, an alternative approach is to lay the child down between your legs (either on the floor or on a bed), then wrap your legs atop their own, and allow your partner to gently restrain their hands as you support their head while brushing.

Should I be using toothpaste or just brush with water at this age?

Even at this young age, you should absolutely be using a toothpaste that contains fluoride. Tooth-brushing works in two ways. First, the mechanical act of brushing physically removes food and bacteria off the teeth. Second, the exposure to fluoride strengthens the enamel, making it more resistant to decay. Here's a pro tip—make sure the flavor of the toothpaste is agreeable to your child. Many children do not do enjoy "spicier" flavors like mint or cinnamon as much as they do mild fruitier flavors. The more your child enjoys the brushing experience, the easier it will be for both parties.

What is fluoride?

Fluoride is a naturally occurring mineral derived from the element fluorine. It has been successfully used in the United States as an effective means of preventing and controlling the development of dental cavities since the 1940s.

How does fluoride work?

Fluoride works in a number of ways to help make teeth more resistant to decay. *Topical fluorides*, like those found in toothpastes, mouthwashes, and varnishes, work to strengthen the surface of a tooth by incorporating the mineral into the enamel's crystalline structure. These topical fluorides can also have an antibacterial effect by helping to shutdown acid production—and less acid means fewer cavities. In addition to preventing new cavities, topical fluoride therapies may also slow or even reverse the earliest signs of decay, known as *decalcification*. Topical fluorides are most effective with frequent exposure to small amounts, just as you would get from brushing twice daily. It is also important for children to ingest small amounts of *systemic fluorides* via tap water or prescription tablets because the body uses the mineral as a building block to strengthen the teeth that are still forming under the gums.

Is fluoride safe?

When used appropriately, fluoride is safe and effective in preventing and controlling dental cavities.[11] The American Dental Society, the American Academy of Pediatrics, the U.S. Public Health Service, and the World Health Organization all endorse the use of fluoridated water. In fact, nearly all medical, dental, and public health organizations recommend the use of fluoride. There has been no scientific evidence linking community water fluoridation at appropriate levels with any potential adverse health risks.[12] In the United States, community water fluoridation was named "one of the top ten greatest public health achievements of the twentieth century" by the Center for Disease Control and Prevention (CDC).[13]

How do I know if my tap water has fluoride in it?

According to the CDC, the optimal fluoride level in water is 0.7 milligrams per liter. You can obtain information about water fluoridation in your area by contacting your local water utility provider. Their contact details are usually located on your water bill. If your home gets water from a well, most local well companies can test the water for fluoride, as is often done on a home inspection. The CDC website also has a helpful section called "My Water's Fluoride (MWF)" that allows you to look up the water fluoridation status of your local area. Type "CDC MWF" into your online search engine and follow the appropriate prompts. Your dentist may also be knowledgeable about local fluoridation water status, so don't be afraid to ask questions.

If my home water supply is not fluoridated, do I need to get supplements?

Your dentist, or pediatrician, may consider prescribing supplements for your child after reviewing their total dietary fluoride intake and their individual *risk factors* for developing cavities. Even though a child may not be getting fluoride from local tap water, they may still be getting it from other sources, including infant formula or foods produced in areas using fluoridated water. As a general rule, most infants under six-months of age should not receive prescription fluoride supplements regardless of the fluoride content in their water. Children between the ages of six-months to three-years could benefit from a low dose of fluoride.[14] You should check with your dentist to see if your child falls into the at-risk category.

Do I need to buy special children's toothpaste?

No, you don't. While children's toothpaste will often have lower percentages of fluoride and different flavors, like bubblegum, to make them more agreeable to kids, any over-the-counter toothpaste is fine when used as instructed. For a young child, aged zero to three, the caregiver should place only a thin film of toothpaste, called a "smear," on the brush head. This smear should be no larger than a grain of rice.[14] The small amount will provide the benefits of cavity protection while minimizing the amount of paste the child could potentially swallow. After brushing, wipe away any excess toothpaste with a clean cloth.

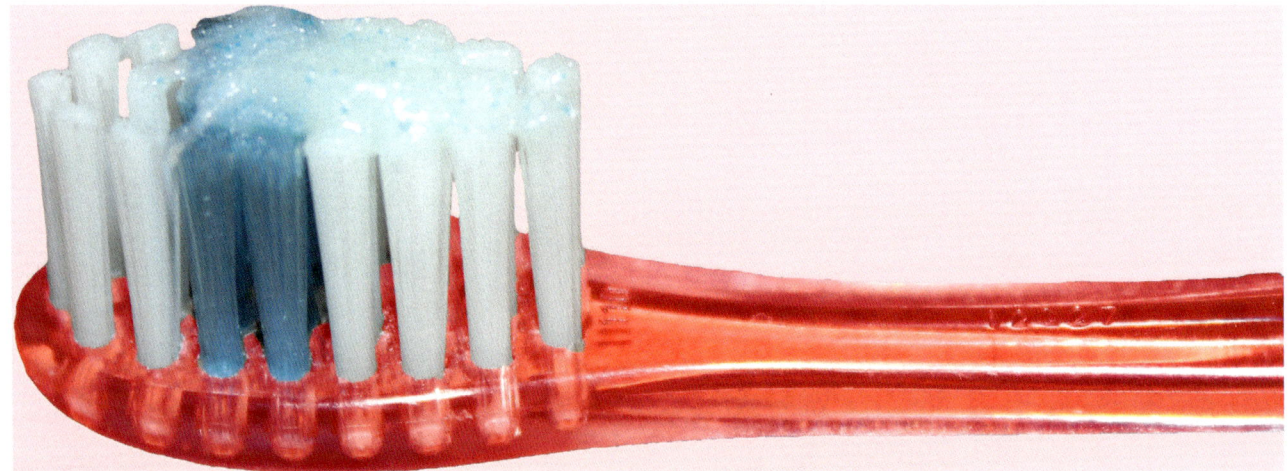

Smear amount of toothpaste seen on children's toothbrush.

What if my child swallows toothpaste?

If your child does swallow the small smear used while brushing, there is no need to worry. However, if they find a way to ingest a large or unknown quantity of toothpaste, call your dentist or poison control immediately. The first symptom is generally gastrointestinal discomfort, but headache, tremors, and alterations to vision are also possible. It is often recommended to give your child milk or yogurt to prevent an upset stomach as the calcium in these foods helps to trap the fluoride. Inducing vomiting in these situations is not recommended unless specifically directed by a physician or poison control.[15]

My child received fluoride varnish at their last dental visit. What is that about?

A *varnish* is a professionally applied sticky fluoride-containing material that is painted on the teeth, usually after a cleaning, to prevent or slow the progression of cavities. Due to their favorable characteristics, varnishes are the standard for in-office fluoride therapies. They have higher fluoride concentrations than available over-the-counter products. They can be applied quickly, making them great for use with children or uncooperative patients. Their sticky nature allows them to adhere to teeth, increasing the duration of contact and preventing the child from swallowing excessive amounts of the material. After its application, it is recommended not to eat or drink for thirty-minutes.

When do I need to start flossing?

Flossing is important because the bristles on a toothbrush cannot thoroughly clean the small spaces where teeth touch one another. These tight areas are known as *contacts* and they are very prone to getting cavities. At this age however, most children will have open spaces between their teeth and lack the aforementioned contacts. Spaces between the teeth confer a number of advantages: they make the teeth more cleansable by the child's own saliva and tongue, toothbrush bristles can reach the sides of teeth more easily, and debris are less prone to becoming entrapped in the contact area. With that said, flossing becomes necessary once teeth are in close proximity and touch their neighbors. Let's make it simple—if teeth are touching, you should be flossing.

Does breastfeeding affect my child's teeth?

The benefits of breastfeeding have been well established during a child's first year of life. It is a source of nutrients, immune system mediators, and a means of bonding. However, breastfeeding beyond twelve-months of age, especially if done frequently and/or at nighttime, is associated with the development of cavities in early childhood.[16]

How should I clean my child's mouth after breastfeeding?

Consider wiping your child's gums, or teeth if they have them, with a clean washcloth after each feeding. For children with teeth, this intermittent cleaning is done in addition to the twice-daily brushes.

Are there any "no-nos" in regard to baby bottles?

Infants who are bottle-feeding should **never** be put to sleep with their bottle, particularly if it contains milk, formula, or juice. Notice how the "never" is in bold lettering—that's how important this is. Putting children to sleep with a bottle permits prolonged bathing of the teeth in sugars that can lead to cavities and a pattern of dental decay known as *baby bottle rot*. Weaning from the bottle should be encouraged by twelve-months of age in favor of an open cup.[17] Avoiding this big mistake may be the single most important thing you can do to help your infant stave off getting dental cavities.

Why is an open cup preferred over a "sippy" cup?

Similar to bottles, covered "sippy" cups essentially enable children to nurse their drinks for extended periods of time. The amount of time teeth are exposed to sugars is directly linked to the development of cavities. Time, not overall quantity, is the key factor here. Open cups encourage children to finish their drinks over a set time interval rather than allowing them the convenience to keep coming back for more and more sugar exposures.

Is juice healthy?

Juices are almost never a good option for kids, especially when compared to alternative fluids such as milk and water. Juices lack the healthy fibers that whole fruits and vegetables contain, and the vitamins that juice companies tout can be obtained through a healthy diet alone.[18] Juices contain natural sugars and acids that, when combined with bacterial acids in the mouth, can create a potent cocktail for the formation of cavities. The American Academy of Pediatrics recommends that children under one year of age not receive any juice unless prescribed by a physician, and children of one to three years of age receive at most four ounces in a day. Let's be absolutely clear on the matter—forgo the juice for water.

If my child does get a cavity in a baby tooth, why bother fixing it? Won't it just fall out anyway?

This is one of the most common misconceptions we hear as dentists. A cavity is a byproduct of bacteria and the result of an *infection*. In the early stages, this infection is confined to only the outer layers of the tooth. If the problem is ignored, cavities grow and infiltrate deeper until they reach the innermost layer called the *pulp*. From the pulp, we are "off to the races," as the infection can quickly travel through the roots to the jawbones that hold the teeth in place. Here in the jaws, the adult teeth are developing, and an infection in this area can damage them while they are in their fragile state. Once the infection has spread beyond the tooth and into the bone, pus can accumulate and we likely will see an *abscess* or *facial swelling* develop. Remember that everything in the body is interconnected and a swelling in the mouth could easily spread down to the child's neck or up to their eyes and potentially their brain. Children are frequently admitted to hospitals due to neglected dental cavities that can lead to life threatening infections.[19] Don't risk it...it is very important to treat cavities, even in baby teeth!!!

What happens if my child chips a tooth at this age?

Chipping a tooth is a very common occurrence in this age group, especially a front tooth. Young children are uncoordinated, still learning to walk, and are prone to minor accidents and falls. A minor chip involving only the outer enamel can often be left alone. If the tooth is symptomatic, jagged enough to injure the child's tongue or lips, or if the tooth is displaced, a consultation with your dentist should be pursued as soon as possible.

What happens if the tooth is broken in half?

If a baby tooth is injured to the point where a significant portion of its structure is lost, the tooth will require professional intervention. This treatment may include a possible filling or crown. In the event that the pulp is exposed, as evidenced by a pink or red dot at the center of the tooth, the baby tooth in question may require an extraction. Contact your dentist for a full work-up in this situation.

What if an accident has pushed a tooth out of alignment?

Compared to adults, children's bones are more pliable, and so quite frequently an accident that would otherwise break an adult tooth might instead displace a baby tooth out of position. This type of injury is called a *luxation*. It is advisable to contact your dental professional, as the treatment will depend on the direction and severity of the luxation. Often these injuries are managed conservatively, by allowing the tooth to spontaneously make its way back into the proper position. However, more severe injuries, or those that pose a risk to the developing adult teeth, may be better addressed with extractions.

Should I be concerned with too much thumb sucking or pacifier use?

These habits are relatively common at this age, providing a means of security and self-soothing. Though long-term negative dental consequences of thumb sucking (detailed in Chapters 4 and 9) are not typically seen if the habit stops by age three, the sooner one can stop the better. Most children will stop these habits all on their own.

What is a tongue-tie?

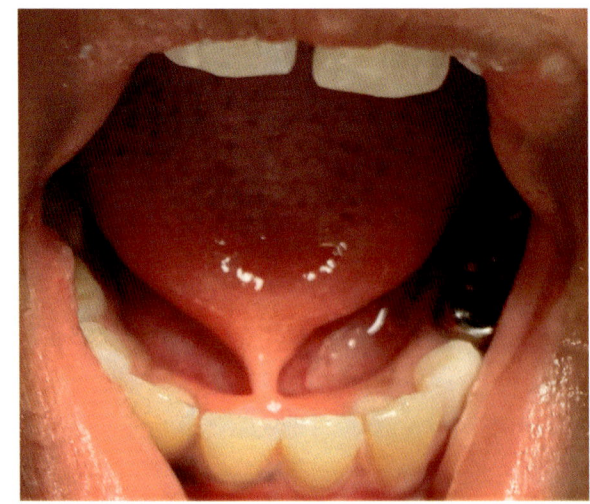

A tongue-tie, more formally known as *ankyloglossia*, is an anomaly characterized by an abnormally short, thick, or tight band of tissue connecting the tongue to the lower gums. Most babies are checked for tongue-ties early in life, and they are reported in 4 to 10 percent of newborns.[20,21,22] Pediatricians, dentists and lactation consultants are all on the lookout for these.

How do I know if I need to get a tongue-tie fixed?

According to the American Academy of Pediatric Dentistry, "No universally accepted criteria has been established for making this diagnosis. Most systems rely on a combination of anatomic and functional markers." In other words, tongue-ties are diagnosed if and when the child has associated problems with the movement and functioning of their tongue. Appearance alone is not an indication for tongue-tie surgery. Some of these issues include breast- or bottle-feeding difficulties, speech impairments, poor alignment of teeth, and gingival recession (a condition where the gums migrate downward toward the root).

My newborn has white/yellow patches on their tongue and palate. What is that?

These patches are likely to be *oral thrush*, caused by a fungal species known as *Candida*. Fungi are normal inhabitants of the oral cavity, yet we typically don't see overt signs of their colonization in most children and adults. Infants, however, are at heightened risk for this fungal overgrowth since their immune system is immature and not yet firing on all cylinders. Infants who have taken antibiotics are even more susceptible to developing thrush. These drugs can wipe out the natural bacteria in the mouth, allowing the fungi to multiply and establish themselves in their place.

How do I treat thrush?

Mild cases can potentially clear up on their own. In moderate to severe cases, your doctor or dentist may prescribe a topical *anti-fungal* agent to be used for approximately one week. It is also good practice to boil and disinfect foreign objects like pacifiers, bottle nipples, or toys that your child puts in their mouth. Consult your physician if you are currently breastfeeding a child with thrush to discuss potentially modifying their feeding routine.

My child has a significant number of sores in and around their mouth. What should I do?

For a child in this age group, one of the most common reasons for the sudden appearance of numerous mouth sores is a condition known as *Primary Herpetic Gingivostomatitis*. This is a fancy name used to describe the first breakout of the *Herpes Simplex Virus* in your child. Approximately 10 to 30 percent of children will display this initial outbreak, and many more will acquire the virus but simply never show signs of the infection.[23,24] Typically, a child's gums will appear red, swollen, and numerous *vesicles* (fluid-filled blisters) will crop up in and around the mouth. Shortly after they first appear, these blisters will rupture and become painful craters called *ulcers*. Other symptoms may include fever, malaise, irritability, trouble eating (due to discomfort), and swollen lymph nodes. Treatment usually involves making sure the child stays hydrated and administering over-the-counter pain relievers and anti-fever drugs to control the discomfort. Mild cases will typically take about seven to ten days for the lesions and symptoms to disappear.

If my child has herpes sores, are they contagious?

Yes. It is important to note that herpes lesions are contagious and your child may share the virus with others, including siblings, other children, and even adults who were never infected.[25] The risk of transmission is greatest when active blisters and sores are present, but the virus can be spread at any time. During the initial breakout, it is prudent to keep the child home from school or daycare to minimize exposing others to the virus.

"You may delay, but time will not."
– Benjamin Franklin

The early years are a crucial period that sets the tone for your child's smile story. We hope you will embrace this opportunity to get them started on the right track to oral health. Early prevention and intervention are the takeaways in this age group. Build a foundation of good hygiene habits, watch their diet, and find yourself a dentist who will partner with you to help guide their smile in the years to come.

CHAPTER 4
AGE THREE TO SIX – MOLAR MILESTONES

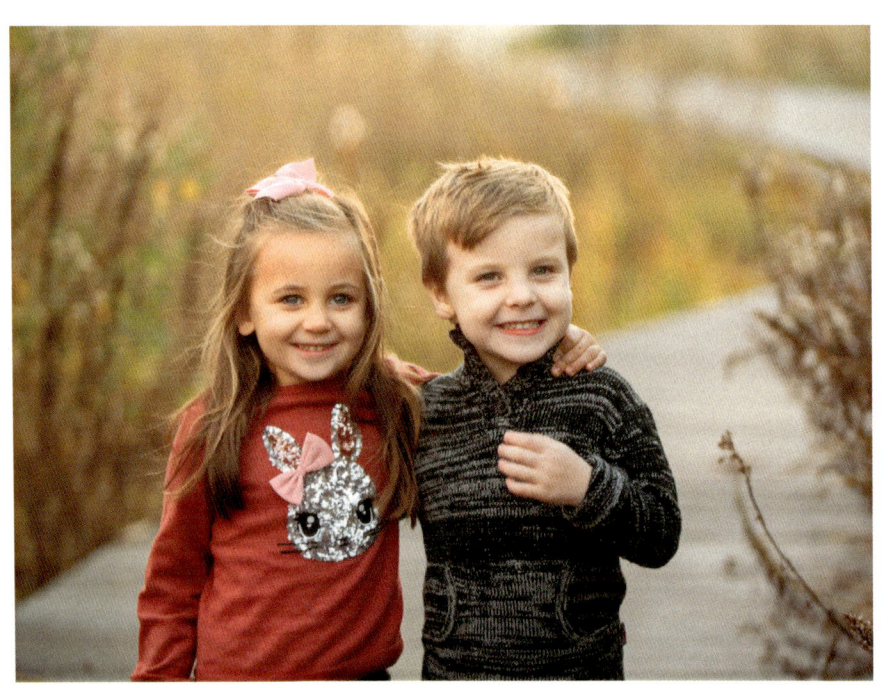

Kids of this age group tend to be a lot of fun. They start to make friends, tell stories, and use their imagination to play pretend. They are also sponges of information and have an urge to discover the world around them. As a parent, you will be your child's first teacher, leading them on this journey of discovery. Whether it's learning the rules of addition or how to tie their shoes, it's important to provide them guidance and support in these endeavors. The same is true in regard to their dental habits—teach them the rules of oral health. Preschool aged children tend to enjoy being good helpers, thriving off the boundaries you set for them, and seeking to gain your approval by following instructions. Lean into their desire to learn and please, encourage them, and acknowledge them for a job well done.

How many teeth should be in the mouth by age three?

Typically, all twenty of the baby teeth are in the mouth by age three. Dentists will often use this age as a checkpoint to ensure that things are progressing according to plan.

Is it possible to have more or less than twenty baby teeth?

Yes, it's entirely possible. Approximately 1 percent of children may be missing some baby teeth, known as *hypodontia,* or be born with extra baby teeth, known as *hyperdontia*.[26] It is also possible to have two teeth fused together, forming one larger-than-normal sized tooth. In most cases, these anomalies are just random findings, but in some rare cases, they can be evidence of an underlying medical condition.

What should be happening in the mouth between the ages of three and six?

There are few visible dental changes that occur during this time. Most of the action is happening underneath the gums with the development of the permanent teeth and changes to the size of the facial structure and jawbones.

What can happen to the adult teeth developing at this age?

Just as the primary teeth were once susceptible to damage while in utero, so too are the permanent teeth now in their fragile state of development beneath the gums. Significant childhood illnesses, vitamin deficiencies, and infections of the baby teeth can damage the adult teeth, causing them to be malformed, misaligned, or discolored. We call teeth that have experienced defects during their development *hypoplastic*.

How often should my child be going to the dentist for routine care?

Following your first dental visit, your child should be seen at least twice annually for routine preventative check-ups. Note that for children who are at higher risk of getting cavities, the frequency of dental visits may be higher, such as every three-months rather than twice a year. The additional visits enable the dental team to keep a closer eye on things to intercept developing problems before they grow in size and severity.

How might a routine dental visit change for a three to six-year-old?

Around the age of three to four, most children will feel comfortable enough separating from their parents to sit in the dental chair by themselves. They should be able to follow simple directions from the dental team, such as open, close, swallow, and smile. Now is also the age that many dentists will start taking radiographs, commonly called X-rays, on your children's teeth.

Are X-rays really necessary so soon?

The need for X-rays on any child should be determined on an individualized basis. While X-rays are used primarily by your dentist to detect cavities that cannot be seen by the naked eye, they may also be used to evaluate growth and development. In particular, your dentist will be looking at the number of forming adult teeth and checking the bones of the jaw for irregular findings.

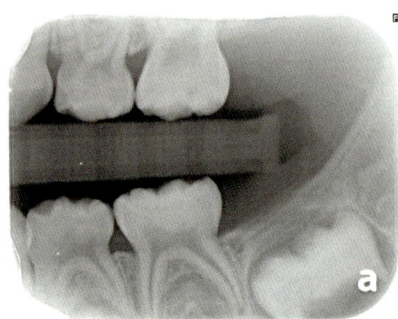

X-rays known as *bitewings* at age three.

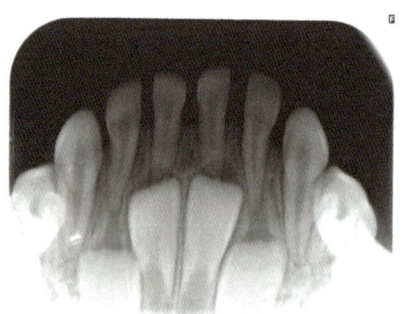

X-rays known as *occlusals* at age three.

How frequently should my child get X-rays?

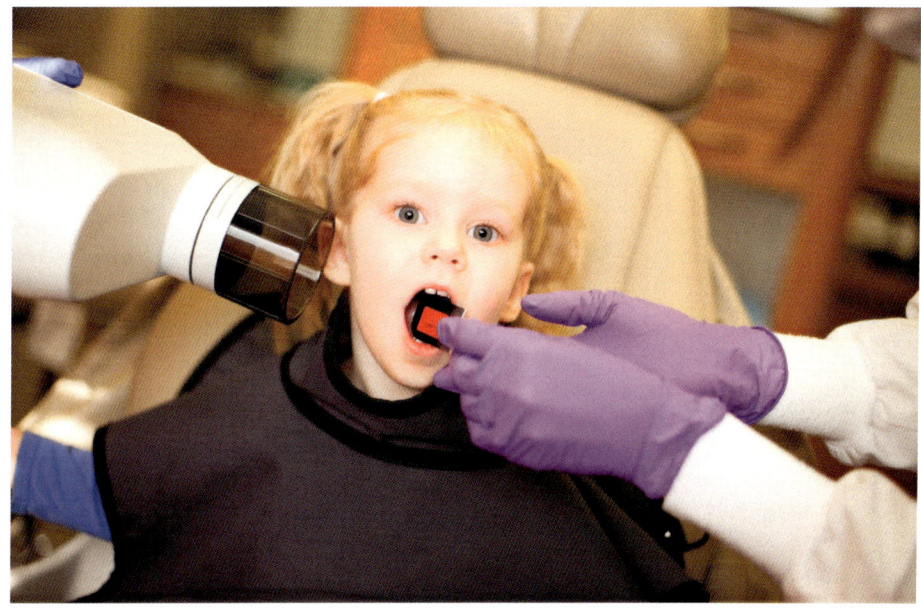

There is no one-size-fits-all answer to this question. You should expect that most clinicians will want an initial set of X-rays to establish a baseline of your child's dental health. From there, the frequency of "routine" X-rays should depend on the child's risk of developing new cavities. A high-risk child, one who may have had cavities in the past, or appears to have poor dietary or hygiene habits, may need X-rays to be taken every six-months. However, a child who has never shown signs of dental disease and appears to have good home care, may only need X-rays to be taken every twenty-four months.

Are dental X-rays safe for my developing child?

Some people worry about dental X-rays because they work by exposing our bodies to a small amount of *radiation*. While this is a true statement, it is also true that there are much more significant sources of radiation all around us in our daily lives. The majority of radiation we receive annually comes from natural sources, including the ground, the foods we eat, and cosmic rays from outer space. Depending on where you live, your activities, and your frequency of travel, your daily exposure varies greatly. Take airplane travel for example. The amount of radiation exposure on a flight from New York City to Los Angeles is equivalent to 200 single-tooth X-rays![27] If you are curious about what types of radiation exposures you or your child may have day-to-day, check out The American Nuclear Society's website. They have a "Dose Calculator." The link can be found in the helpful links section in the back of the book.

Dental X-rays by comparison are *very low-dose* radiation exposures and present only a minimal risk to the patient. That small risk is far outweighed by the risk of not taking X-rays and missing disease. Dentists will use additional safeguards such as thyroid collars and high-speed digital films to further reduce the amount of radiation the child will receive. The goal is to expose your child to the lowest possible amount of radiation while obtaining the necessary information to diagnose problems.

Is it still normal to still have spaces between baby teeth?

Yes, it is normal and usually considered a good thing to have these spaces. The forthcoming adult teeth will be considerably wider than the baby teeth they will replace; they will need this extra space when trying to fit into the dental arch. It is also common to see larger than average gaps, known as *primate spaces*, between the upper lateral incisors and canines, and the lower canines and first molars. These primate spaces will help a great deal to accommodate for the discrepancy of tooth sizes.

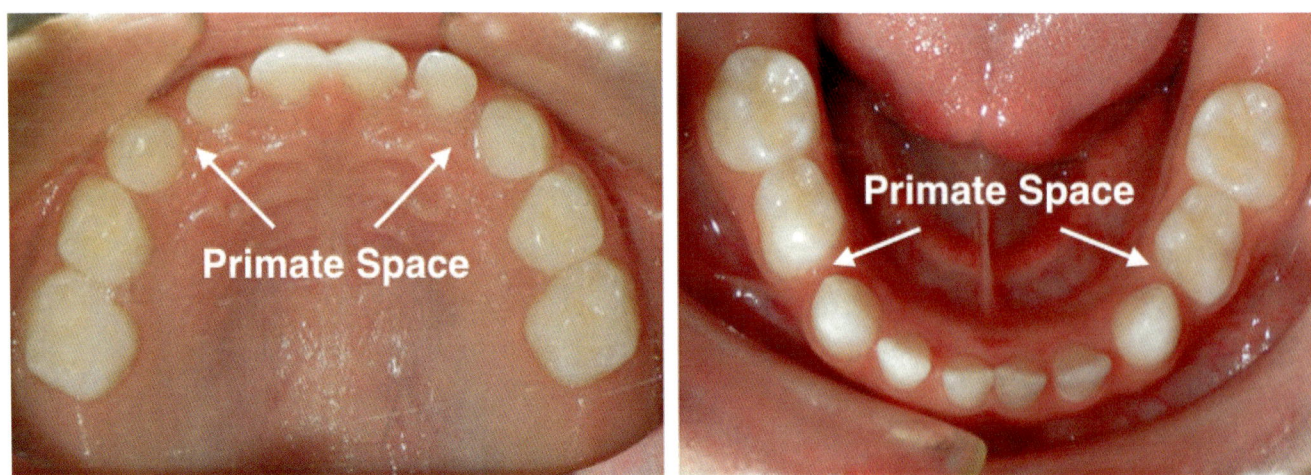

Primate spacing on a four-year-old (upper teeth left, lower teeth right)

How important is it to maintain baby teeth?

It is vital to maintain your child's baby teeth. Not only do they help us chew, speak, and smile, but they also have the important job of guiding the adult teeth to their final positions. Baby teeth essentially act as placeholders for the adult teeth that will follow them. If we lose a baby tooth too early, the corresponding adult tooth may come into the wrong position, or not have enough room to erupt at all. For all these reasons, we want to preserve our baby teeth until they naturally fall out at the appropriate time. With a focus on good oral hygiene, a healthy diet, and preventative care—you can help your child maintain their baby teeth until the time is right.

How should we be brushing at this age?

With all the baby teeth in the mouth, you should now be placing a "pea-sized" amount of toothpaste on the brush rather than the thin smear that was suggested in the last chapter.[28] With continued growth and development, it is also possible that the back teeth are now contacting one another. Remember, if teeth are touching adjacent teeth, it's time to start flossing between them—do this at least once daily.

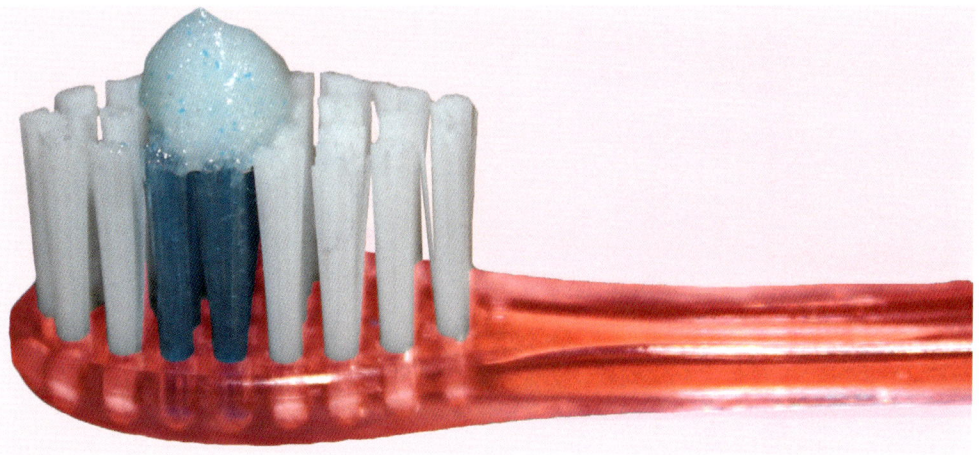

The proper amount of toothpaste for this age.

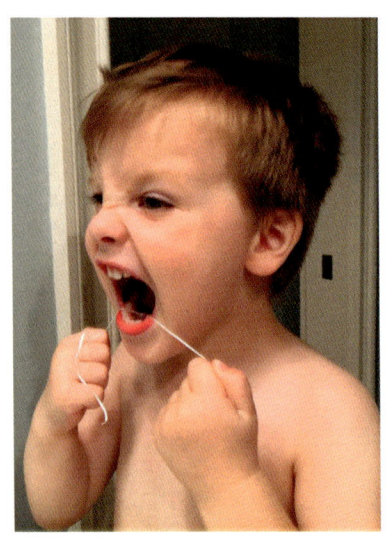

Many children in this age group will wish to demonstrate independence and attempt brushing themselves. While parents should encourage this initiative, they should also keep in mind that the child's motor skills, and therefore their ability to do a good job brushing, are still questionable at best. Children left unsupervised may only brush for a matter of seconds and consider the job sufficiently done. So, our best recommendation for this age group is to allow children the opportunity to first brush their own teeth, let them feel a sense of self-accomplishment, and then have the parent follow-up with a second round of high-quality brushing for two-minutes twice daily.

Should I get my child an electric toothbrush or are the old-fashioned ones fine?

Both electric (battery-powered) and manual brushes do an adequate job of removing plaque and debris when used appropriately. Therefore, use whichever brush will motivate your child the most. There's a plethora of options out there with different colors, cartoon characters, and some that even time their brushing with music… just go with the flow and embrace your child's enthusiasm. Regardless of the style you choose, be careful that you or your child are not applying too much force while brushing, as excessive pressure can cause irritation and damage to the teeth and gums if done repeatedly.

"I will brush my teeth good, so they can be like a lion. ROAR!"

– Leora, five years old

What about mouthwashes?

First and foremost, mouthwashes are not a substitute for an adequate brushing and flossing routine. Secondly, young children, especially those under six-years of age, are at risk of swallowing large quantities of mouthwash relative to their body size and should therefore only be using them under the direct supervision of a parent when prescribed to do so by a dentist. Over-the-counter mouthwashes may contain alcohol (in the form of ethanol), which can lead to serious side effects in children if swallowed. It is strongly recommended to avoid these alcohol-containing products in this age group entirely.

Why is my child afraid of going to the dentist?

Your child is not alone. Many factors may be at play in this age group. These include fear of strangers, fear of the unknown, fear of strange instruments, new and uncomfortable sensations in the mouth, and unusual or loud sounds. Language and terminology can also scare children who do not know their meaning. Children are also typically unable to view what is happening in their mouth as the dentist works, and they may not know to trust the doctor yet. These fears can be grounded in reality from previous negative experiences or acquired vicariously from peers or familial anxiety.

How can I help reduce my child's fear of going to the dentist?

We have already discussed the first important step in setting your child up for success—getting them used to visiting the dentist from a young age. Secondly, children learn from their parents. They listen to the language you use, and they notice the anxieties you project. Now is not the time to share your own fears and "horror stories" from your childhood experiences. Even if you, as an adult, do not like going to the dentist, you need to pretend you enjoy it for the sake of your child. It is best to talk to your child about the upcoming appointment and *frame it in a positive light*. For example, you can say, "A dentist is someone who counts your teeth and makes sure they are healthy and strong." That sounds a lot better than "The dentist is going to check you for cavities." To a child, a statement like that can provoke substantial fear. They may think, "What's a cavity? What are they going to do to me if they find one?"

The dentist should never be used as a threat. Avoid telling your child that they'll get "shots" and "needles" in their mouth as a punishment for poor brushing and/or snacking habits. Do not use words like "hurt," "drill," and "pulling teeth" when describing potential treatments. We recommend using age appropriate terms whenever possible. For example, instead of saying "bacteria" to a four-year-old, we would suggest saying "sugar bugs." Instead of "getting an extraction," a better alternative would be "making a gift for the tooth fairy."

If your child is in this age group and has yet to go to the dentist, consider doing a rehearsal visit at home first. The parent plays the role of the doctor, and instructs their child to sit back in a chair while they count and brush their teeth in the same manner a dentist would. The closer you can simulate the experience of going to the dentist's office, the more practiced and less nervous they will be during the real thing. Numerous picture books and videos are also available to demonstrate to kids what to expect in a non-threatening manner.

Opinions vary, but we also recommend not bribing your child to behave at the dentist. While this may work on some children, consider for yourself why someone would bribe you into doing something… the task must not be that pleasant if it takes a bribe for you to agree to it. Many children are smart enough to figure this out. Do, however, *positively reinforce* children after they have done well to strengthen the desired behavior. This can be with verbal praise or a physical gift for a job well done!

What should I do if my child develops a toothache?

Your best course of action is to make an appointment with your dentist to address the underlying issue. In the interim, minor toothaches can be managed with over-the-counter pain relievers like ibuprofen or acetaminophen. Topical numbing medications that contain the active ingredient benzocaine are not advised in very young children due to the risk of developing a fatal blood disorder.[29] Consult your dentist or pediatrician to ensure there are no contraindications to these medicines for your child before you introduce them.

My three- to six-year-old fell and damaged their teeth. What do I do?

Take a breath and try not to panic and worry your child further. Instead, remain calm and assess the situation and degree of injury. Some injuries can appear worse than they really are. It is always advisable to contact a medical professional, dentist or pediatrician, when significant trauma events like a bad fall occur. You should keep in mind that all tooth and mouth injuries are really a subset of head injuries, which can be quite serious. If you notice signs of a concussion, they should be discussed with a doctor immediately. Some signs include dizziness, headaches, changes in vision, or vomiting. Children should be evaluated not only for damage to the teeth but also for injuries to the lips, gums, jaws and facial bones. When presented with an injury, your child's dentist will perform an exam and take X-rays to evaluate the full extent of the trauma. In the following example, a four-year-old fell while at summer camp. The injury appeared quite pronounced with bleeding and swelling in the area. The parents were quite distressed and caught up in the commotion of the accident. But were the teeth actually damaged? A trip to the local dental office was very important to thoroughly check the injury. In this case, despite the scary presentation, no fracture or displacement was present and the parents could rest easier knowing the dentist would only need to monitor the teeth over the coming months.

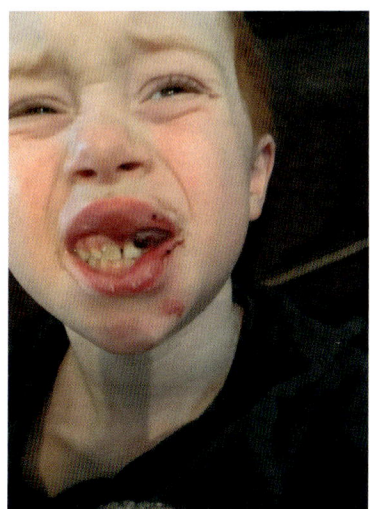

A summer camp accident leading to bleeding and swelling.

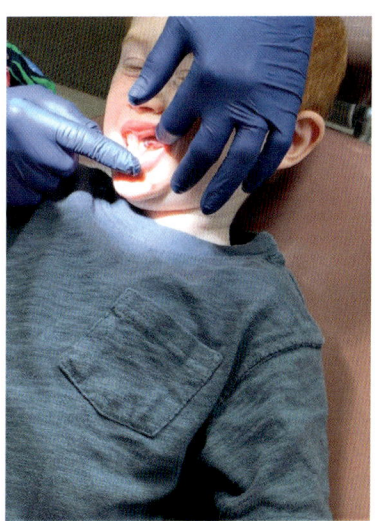

A visit to the dentist to check on the teeth.

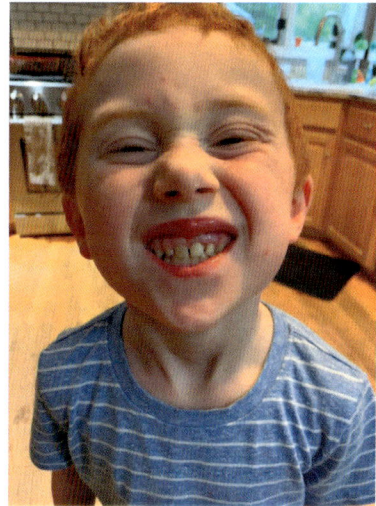

Two weeks later after the swelling had subsided.

What foods are healthy (and unhealthy) for the teeth?

Diet can be complicated in this age range, in part because often as parents we are just focused on getting our picky-eaters to eat anything! Common sense rules apply here. Foods that are healthy for our bodies are also good for our teeth. These include dairy products (milk, yogurt, cheese), proteins (poultry, fish, beans, eggs), and fruits and vegetables. Things that are bad for your teeth are foods and drinks high in sugar and empty calories, such as juices, sodas, and candies. Regardless of what we eat, it is important to clean our teeth afterwards. In an ideal world, we would brush our teeth after having any meal or snack, but since this is not a realistic expectation, simply having water and rinsing your mouth after eating can help decrease the risk of cavities.

What's worse for the teeth: eating a whole bag of chocolates with dinner, or eating only five pieces over the course of an hour?

Well…neither are really good for you. However, when it comes to getting cavities, it's more important to consider how often, and how long, the sugars are in the mouth, rather than just the total amount ingested. A child who *grazes* on carbohydrate-rich foods (like crackers) that will break down into sugars, munching a little here and there, will be worse off in terms of cavity formation than the child who eats the whole bag all at once. This isn't to say that kids can never have candy and snacks, we all deserve to have a little fun from time to time, but whenever possible, consider combining those treats with their three main meals for the day. Frequent snacking is the enemy.

What are some "sneaky" foods that seem healthy but really are not?

We have already touched on the biggest offender—juice. Other snacks that can cause cavities that you might not expect include dried fruits, such as raisins or mango slices. The process of dehydration pulls out the water leaving the remaining fruit more concentrated with sugars and acids. Also, be wary of canned fruits soaking in sugary syrups. Granola bars too can be surprisingly unhealthy, as they can be sticky and sweet, and get stuck in the grooves of the teeth.

My child is still sucking their thumb and/or using a pacifier. Is that bad?

As children get older and continue to suck their thumbs or use pacifiers, negative dental changes will begin to occur. Some common consequences are forward angling of the child's upper front teeth, backward tipping of the bottom front teeth, the development of an *open-bite*, and a narrowing of their palate with potential *crossbite* of the back teeth. We will define and discuss these orthodontic findings in further detail in Chapter 9. The degree to which these negative changes occur depends on the frequency, duration, 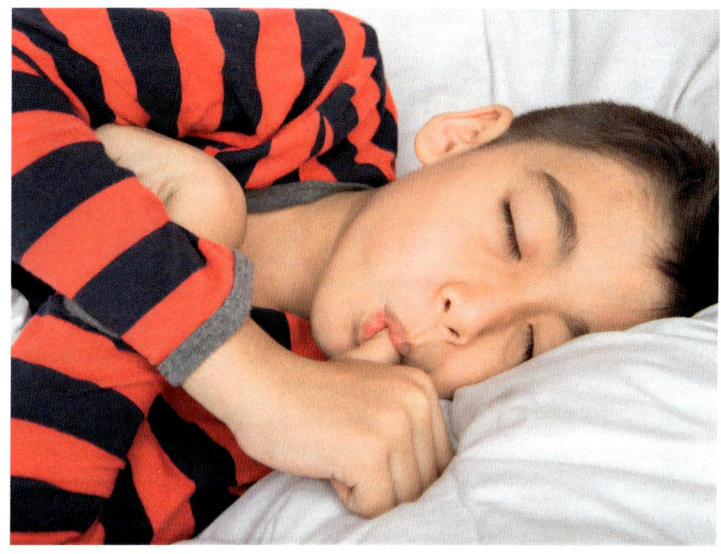 and intensity of the habit. Most children discontinue their sucking behaviors by age four, but for those that do not, it is recommended to try to wean them off these habits before the negative effects start impacting the soon-to-arrive adult teeth.

What can I do to help break my child's sucking habits?

There are a number of techniques you can try. This starts with the basics—simple encouragement and motivation for the child. Use positive reinforcement, rewarding the child every day they make it without having to suck their thumb. If that doesn't work, there are many over-the-counter aids available such as mittens, thumb guards, or bitter solutions to coat the thumb and discourage sucking. If these are still not effective, the dentist may explore more invasive strategies, including placing appliances in the mouth to serve both as a reminder and deterrent of this often involuntary behavior.

How does a dentist fix cavities?

In this age group, we are specifically talking about cavities on baby teeth. Treatment options depend on the number of cavities present, the size of those cavities, the presence or absence of pain, and the child's level of cooperation. After surveying the big picture, the dentist will propose *treatment plans*, which are their best recommendations for care. Small cavities are typically addressed with white-colored fillings that repair part of the tooth. Larger cavities may need crowns, which cover the entirety of the tooth and are available in silver or white color. Teeth with cavities that have become too big to save, or teeth experiencing spontaneous pain, may require extractions.

My child has a swelling from a tooth, why can't I just take antibiotics to fix it?

As we have discussed previously, a cavity is really a sign of a *bacterial infection*. When bacteria start breaking through the hard enamel shell of a tooth, they will eventually reach the inner pulp. The pulp is really the living portion of the tooth. It communicates with the rest of the body by nerves and small blood vessels. Unfortunately, these vessels are so incredibly small that there is insufficient access for antibiotics to really get into the tooth and do the job of cleaning out the infection. Therefore, while the antibiotics might make the swelling go down temporarily, they will never fix the "root" cause of the problem. The bacteria remain in the tooth; they fester, and continue to multiply. Given time, the swelling will inevitably come back if the tooth is not otherwise treated.

My child had a filling done and now their lip looks swollen and infected. What do you think is going on?

The most likely explanation for this problem is *post-anesthesia lip biting*. Anesthetic injections are used by dentists to numb the teeth and remove the sensation of pain before fixing cavities. The lip and tongue are often anesthetized as a side effect of these injections. Some of these numbing medications can last for hours after the procedure is finished. Children, especially young ones, who are unfamiliar with the sensation of numbness may inadvertently bite or chew on themselves in response to the unusual feeling. Only after the numbing medication wears off will they experience the discomfort they have self-inflicted. Depending on how severe and prolonged the biting is, the lip may appear significantly swollen and ulcerated. Prevention is the key here; parents should monitor their children after receiving dental anesthesia to ensure they are not traumatizing their lips.

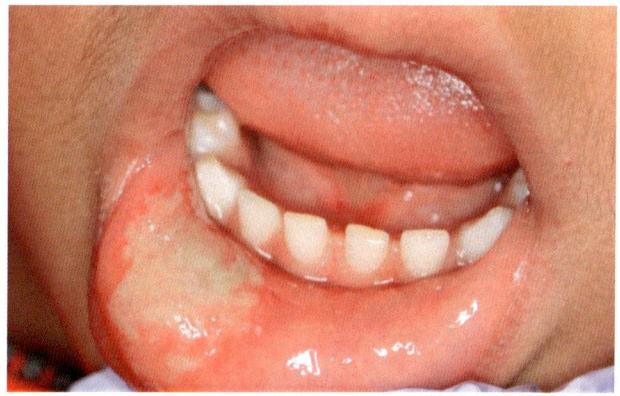

Picture showing a large sore from a child biting on the lip without realization due to anesthesia.

My dentist recommended sedation for my child, what is that about?

Sedation is a technique in which medications are used by dentists to help patients with their anxiety, facilitate cooperation, and reduce the sensation of pain. Typically reserved for cases where there is more involved work such as multiple fillings, extractions, or crowns, sedation allows the dentist to complete high-quality, technique-sensitive work while avoiding certain children's defensive or uncooperative tendencies.

How sedated will my child be? Are they conscious or asleep?

Sedation is a broad term that encompasses multiple levels of *depth*. A mild sedation is something "light." Your child may be given a small drink of medicine or nasal spray to "take the edge off" their anxiety. They remain awake throughout the procedure, but these medications may produce amnesia so children will not remember any unpleasant experience.

Moderate sedation produces a state of drowsiness, where the patient is still conscious, but their cognitive abilities are weakened. They are still awake to hear what you and the dentist are saying, but they lose some of their desire to "put up a fight." This sedation may be achieved through a mix of medicines the child will usually drink at the dentist's office.

Deep sedation is used when either there is extensive work that needs to be done or your child is more significantly uncooperative from the onset. The patient is essentially "sleeping" and they may need airway assistance from time to time to help them breathe better. This level of sedation is usually administered intravenously.

Is sedation safe? I have heard that children have died during dental sedations.

It is true that sedation is not without its risks, and deaths, though exceedingly rare, have unfortunately happened in dental offices in the past. It is the anesthesia provider's responsibility to minimize the potential risks to help keep your child as safe as possible. *Safety protocols* should include an advanced educational background in conducting sedation on the part of the provider, training in basic and pediatric advanced life support, thorough *preoperative assessment* of your child's eligibility for sedation, the use of medications that are appropriately dosed and tailored to need, continuous *monitoring* of the patient's vital signs, and a venue that must have access to emergency equipment, medications, and personnel. Care must also be taken to ensure the child is no longer under the influence of the sedative medications when being sent home; rather they should be alert and similar to their baseline self. When the appropriate precautions are followed, sedations can be performed with a greater degree of predictability and safety. Hundreds of thousands of sedations are performed annually by dentists across the United States, the vast majority of which happen without incident and provide parents and children a means to complete treatment that would otherwise be prohibitively difficult or traumatizing to the patient.

"Still waters run deep."
– Latin proverb

Though few visible changes have happened to your child's smile during this time frame, much has been brewing beneath the seemingly calm surface. Your child has matured from a toddler with a limited grasp of the alphabet, to a preschooler stringing a few sentences together, to a school-aged child capable of telling their own creative tales. The story of their smile has been evolving too, and soon it will experience a momentous change as the adult teeth make their grand debut. If you want pictures of your child with a full set of teeth, now would be a good time for that photoshoot!

CHAPTER 5
AGES SIX TO EIGHT – TOOTH FAIRY FABLES

Who is ready to start first grade? Common themes from this age group include rambunctious playground games, drop-off playdates, and the classic wish of "All I want for Christmas is my two front teeth." It's a thrilling stage of development, especially for the mouth! All the build-up of the last few years has led to this moment, when your child's smile story begins to take a dramatic turn. Like the humble caterpillar poised to transform, a metamorphosis of epic proportions is on the horizon. Just don't expect a beautiful butterfly right away though, their smile will get there eventually, but the transition will take your child's teeth through some awkward looks along the way. Give it time…every ugly duckling becomes a swan.

When do the adult teeth start coming in? Which ones are supposed to be first?

On average, we expect the first adult teeth to start erupting into the mouth at six to seven years of age. You can basically flip a coin as to which teeth will come in first. About half the time the *permanent first molars*, also known as six-year molars, will win the race and break through the gums right behind the last baby teeth. However, quite often, the lower central incisors will beat them to the punch and push out the baby teeth they replace in the front. The natural process of losing a baby tooth is known as *exfoliation*.

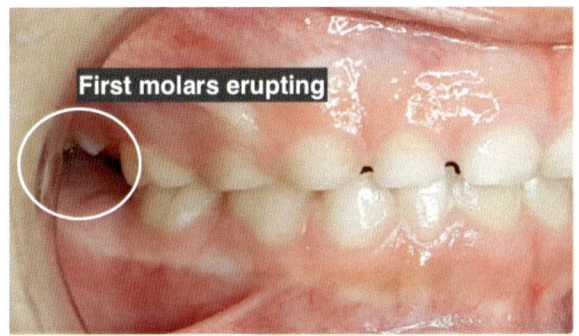 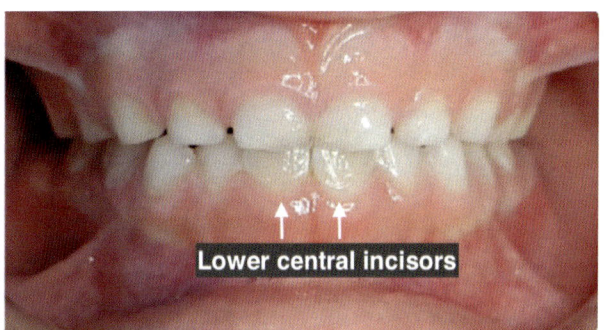

Age Six

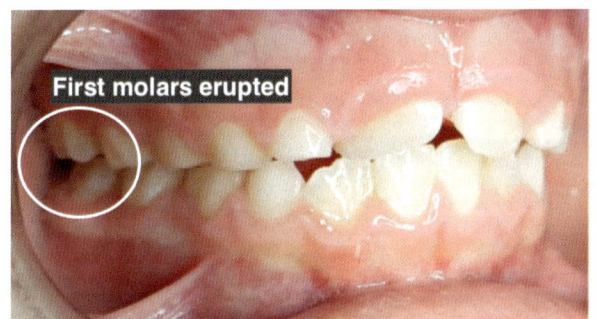 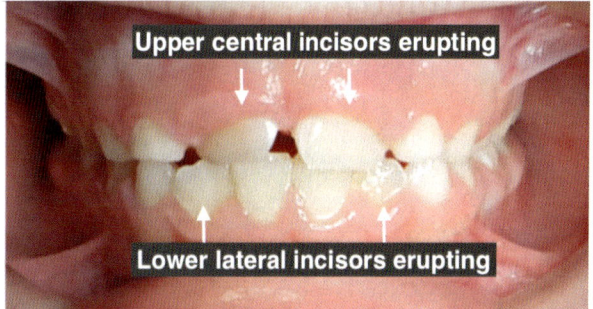

Age Seven

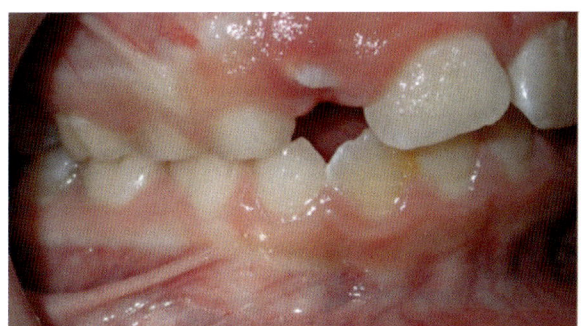 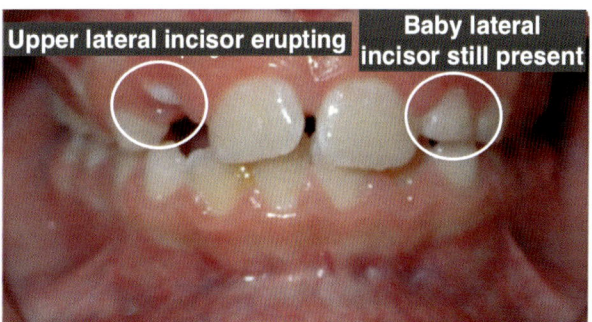

Age Eight

Is there a pattern to the adult teeth erupting?

The basic order of adult teeth coming into the mouth is very similar to the pattern it was for the baby teeth. Typically, the lower teeth will precede the uppers and the sequence will progress from the front to the back of the mouth.

Adult (Permanent) Teeth Chart

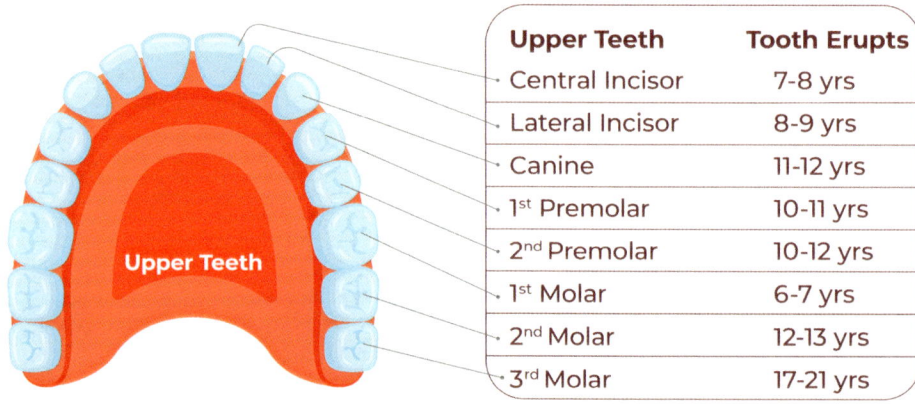

Upper Teeth	Tooth Erupts
Central Incisor	7-8 yrs
Lateral Incisor	8-9 yrs
Canine	11-12 yrs
1st Premolar	10-11 yrs
2nd Premolar	10-12 yrs
1st Molar	6-7 yrs
2nd Molar	12-13 yrs
3rd Molar	17-21 yrs

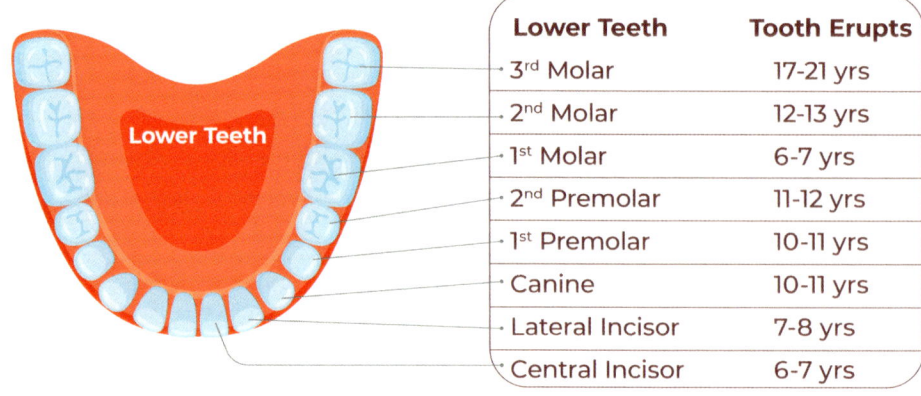

Lower Teeth	Tooth Erupts
3rd Molar	17-21 yrs
2nd Molar	12-13 yrs
1st Molar	6-7 yrs
2nd Premolar	11-12 yrs
1st Premolar	10-11 yrs
Canine	10-11 yrs
Lateral Incisor	7-8 yrs
Central Incisor	6-7 yrs

Is the tooth fairy real?

Sure is…you just need to believe! It's time to embrace the tooth fairy and make losing baby teeth a memorable experience. By this age, most kids are familiar with the tooth fairy through TV, school, or older siblings. Some children will eagerly wiggle out their loose teeth, while others will be nervous and hesitant to do so. Celebrate this milestone by rewarding your child with a small monetary gift, certificate, or even a special toy. The value doesn't matter as much as the joy it brings you and your child. Do your best to turn the experience of losing a tooth, which can sometimes be uncomfortable, into a positive and magical event.

My child is seven-years-old. Is it okay if their front teeth have still not come in yet?

The ages provided are only averages. Just as for baby teeth, there is a lot of variability when it comes to timing. Some kids may experience an accelerated or delayed eruption of their adult teeth without any adverse effects. It is not so much the age, but rather the *sequence* of tooth eruption that is of critical importance. If the wrong adult teeth "cut in line," those teeth may occupy the space intended for other permanent teeth yet to come.

Just how late is too late for their front teeth?

Let us put your mind at ease—healthy children are almost never born missing their front two teeth. In most situations, they just need a little extra time to metaphorically "cook." But, if the central incisors still have not erupted by age eight, it may be worth discussing the concern with your child's dentist, particularly if the lateral incisors are fully in and start using up their space—as this would be a clear example of a sequence problem. In other instances, if the upper central incisors are not in, the lower incisors can continue their path of eruption upwards until they hit the gums where the upper teeth are supposed to go. This pattern can be seen in the accompanying photo of an eight-year-old. The use of X-rays is very important to ensure your child has the correct number of permanent teeth, that they are angled in the proper direction, and that there is nothing blocking their path of eruption.

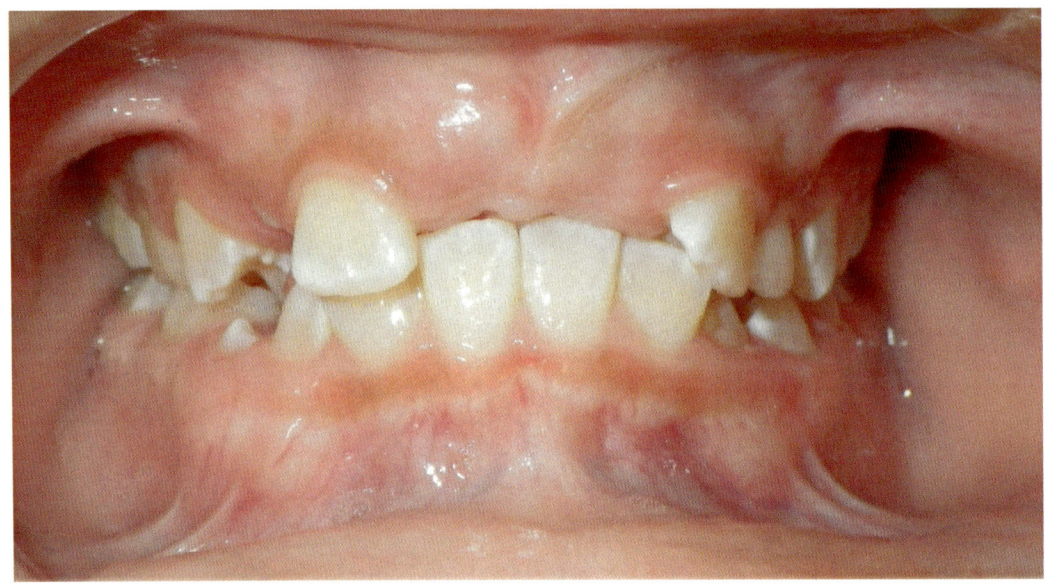

Age Eight – the upper central incisors have not erupted, while the adjacent teeth have. Note the lower incisors have erupted until they are in contact with the gums of the upper central incisors.

What could be blocking teeth from coming in?

There are several reasons a front tooth may not emerge naturally. Perhaps the simplest explanation is *hypertrophic* gum tissue, which is a condition where the gums are thicker or denser than normal, creating resistance for the tooth trying to break through. The solution in this case is simple—a straightforward procedure under local anesthesia to either reduce the gum tissue or expose the tooth usually does the trick. If there isn't enough room for the tooth, some early orthodontic intervention may be warranted to create some space.

Another reason front teeth may be blocked or deflected from coming into the mouth could be the presence of a *mesiodens*, which is an extra tooth present along the middle of the jaw. This extra tooth creates a bit of a traffic jam. Treatment for a mesiodens is typically extraction to remove the blockage. The complexity of removing the tooth depends on the position and orientation of the mesiodens and the teeth around it. An oral surgeon or periodontist most often completes this procedure.

What are the odds my child is missing an adult tooth?

Excluding the central incisors, it's actually much more common for a permanent tooth to be missing compared to a baby tooth. Some studies suggest as many as 9.6 percent of healthy patients are missing one or more adult teeth, and that does not even include the third molars we will discuss in late adolescence.[30] The most commonly missing permanent front tooth is the upper lateral incisor, while the most common back tooth to be missing is the lower second premolar. In addition to the obvious esthetic disadvantages of missing a tooth, the adjacent teeth will often migrate into the empty space, leading to future bite issues.

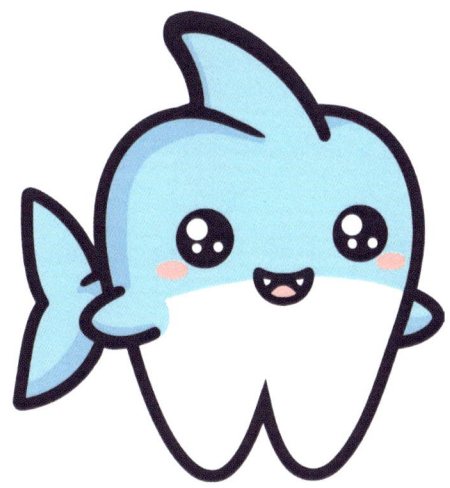

My child's bottom teeth have come in, but the baby teeth have not fallen out. Someone at school called him a shark! What do we do?

It may look a little strange, but rest assured, it is not uncommon for the lower front adult teeth to come into the mouth directly behind the baby teeth that they will eventually replace. This produces a double row of teeth nicknamed "shark teeth." The treatment is often simple and does not require professional intervention—if the baby teeth are already loose, you should encourage your child to wiggle them out, either on their own or with your assistance. Once the baby teeth are gone, the strong muscular force of the tongue will push the permanent teeth forward into proper alignment. However, in some situations, it may be prudent to make an appointment with your dentist to have the baby teeth professionally extracted. This is advisable when the double row has been present for a considerable amount of time (we're talking months), the gap between the two rows of teeth is very large and the baby teeth are not loose at all, or if your child is experiencing pain or inflammation of the gums.

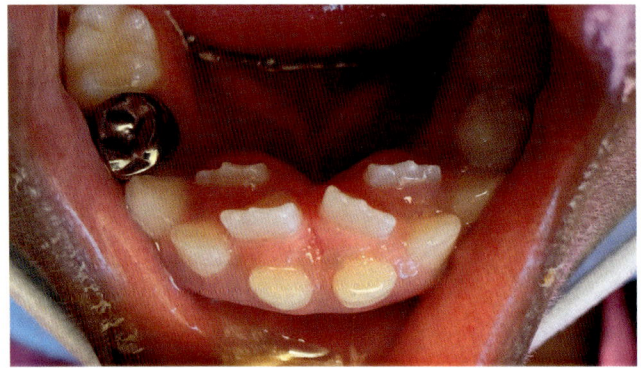

Commonly known as "shark teeth," the lower incisors have erupted behind the baby incisors creating two rows of teeth – like a shark.

One of my child's front teeth came in and looks like a small pointed fang, what is that?

Things in life don't always go according to plan…and sometimes that includes the shape of the teeth! Frequently the upper lateral incisors may develop incorrectly. When these teeth are very small and come to a point, they are referred to as "peg laterals," named after the small wooden pegs they resemble. The treatment for peg lateral incisors involves managing the space around them, and restoring their appropriate size through esthetic procedures such as composite bondings, crowns, or veneers.

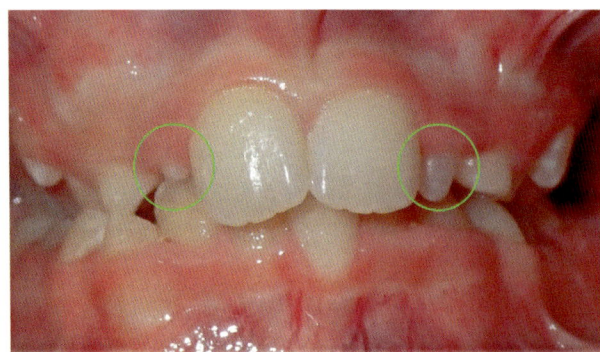

Peg laterals are upper lateral incisors that are smaller than they should be. They often come to a point. There is extensive variation as to how lateral incisors may look as seen in the example above.

If a tooth is dangling, should I wiggle it out or leave it?

If a tooth is so loose that it is dangling, or holding on by a piece of gum tissue, it is best to pull it out. Leaving the tooth there can negatively affect the trajectory of the new tooth trying to come in. Also, bacteria and food debris can become trapped beneath the loose tooth and cause gingival inflammation. Below you can see a baby canine that just did not want to leave on its own—but it was time to send it on its way.

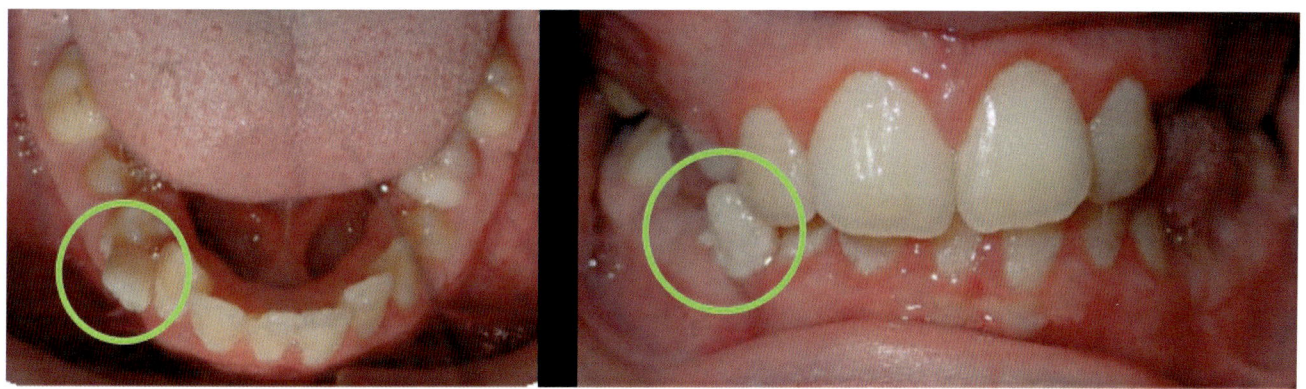

A dangling baby canine, note the gingival inflammation cause by trapped debris.

What are some tips to help wiggle a baby tooth out?

Ultimately, your technique will depend on your child's tolerance and comfort level. While the old tricks like biting into an apple or tying some string around a tooth and doorknob still have their place, often the quickest way to succeed is to simply take your thumb and pointer finger and gently rock the tooth from side to side until it releases from the gums. Parental encouragement and distraction are helpful techniques to get your child through it. Like taking off a bandage, the process may be momentarily uncomfortable, but it's quickly over and done with…and once you're done, you have our permission as a junior dentist to write your child a prescription for their favorite flavor of ice cream.

Why do my child's permanent teeth look so yellow?!

This question is written with both a question mark and an exclamation point at the end of it because it is usually asked with both concern and emotion. Everyone's adult teeth are more yellow and less white than their baby teeth. This contrast of colors is most noticeable in this age group since there is a mix of adult teeth and baby teeth that allows for direct comparison.

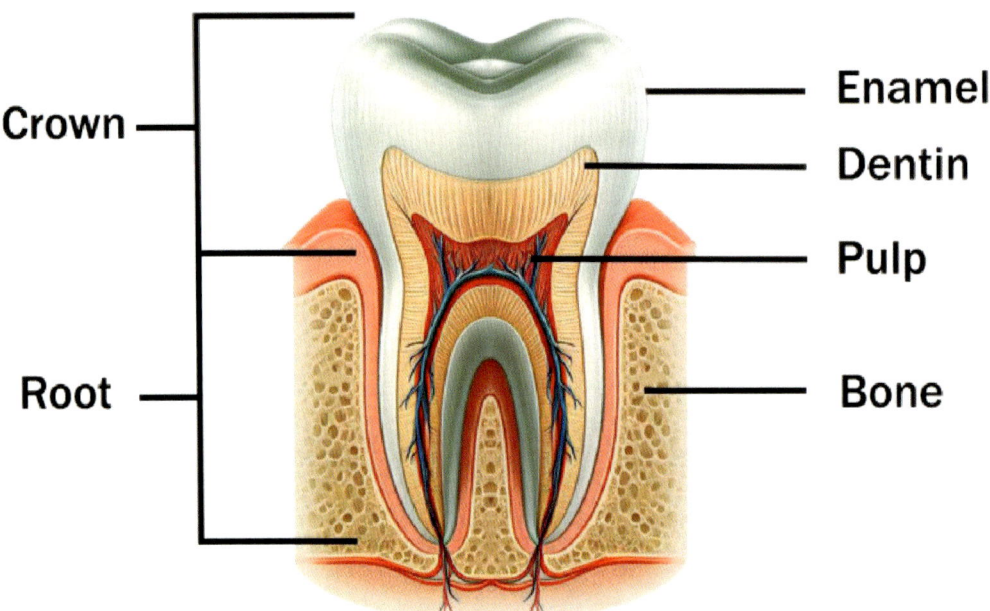

Diagram of the tooth anatomy

Recall that teeth are made up of multiple layers. The outer layer of enamel is relatively translucent. The innermost layer of pulp is reddish-pink due to the presence of blood within it. Sandwiched between these two is a middle layer called *dentin*, which makes up the majority of the tooth and is yellow in color. While both sets of teeth have this yellow dentin, the layer is denser and darker in adult teeth, making them look much yellower by comparison. As your child continues to lose their baby teeth, the color discrepancy between the two sets will become less apparent to the eye.

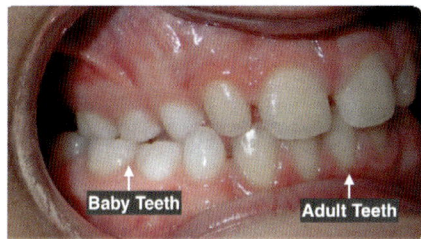 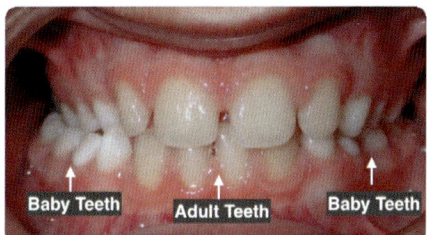 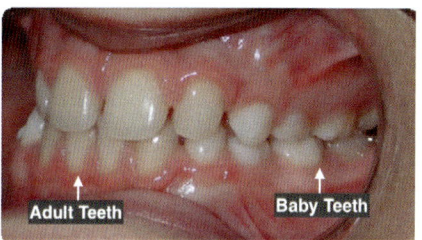

Front permanent teeth are more yellow than the whiter back baby teeth.

My child's front teeth have bumps/ridges on the edges. What are those?

These ridges you see on the edges of your child's incisors are called *mammelons*. They are normal features of these teeth and can be quite prominent. They represent the different developmental sections that merged as the tooth was forming beneath the gums.

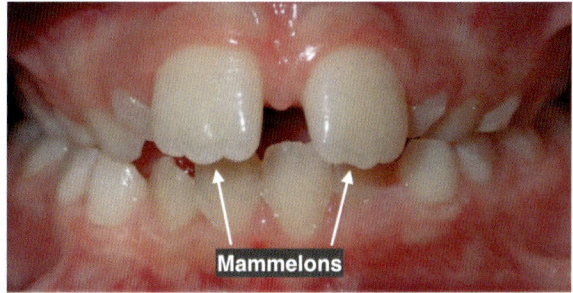 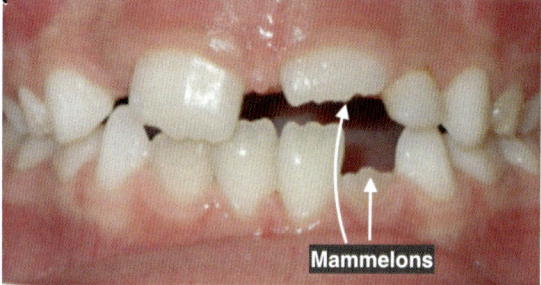

Mammelons are ridges commonly seen on the edges of the front teeth.

Mammelons are at their largest when your child's incisors have just emerged and have yet to reach their final position. Once the top and bottom front teeth begin touching one another, these mammelons will slowly and naturally wear down until the tops of the incisors appear flatter. If over the following years they do not grind down on their own, it may indicate that the front teeth are not touching properly. In such cases, it is advisable to have the issue evaluated by a dentist or orthodontist.

There is a flap of gum tissue over my child's back tooth that is causing discomfort. What is that?

This flap of tissue over a partially erupted tooth is known as an *operculum*. When a molar first breaks through the gums, it initially brings the overlying gingiva with it, covering a portion of the biting surface of the tooth. As the molar erupts further into the mouth, this flap will gradually recede until it is gone completely. Unfortunately, as long as the operculum lies atop the molar, children can very easily bite into and injure it, causing inflammation, ulceration, and considerable pain. Additionally, this flap forms a not-so-nice little pocket that can trap food and bacteria underneath it, further contributing to swelling and discomfort.

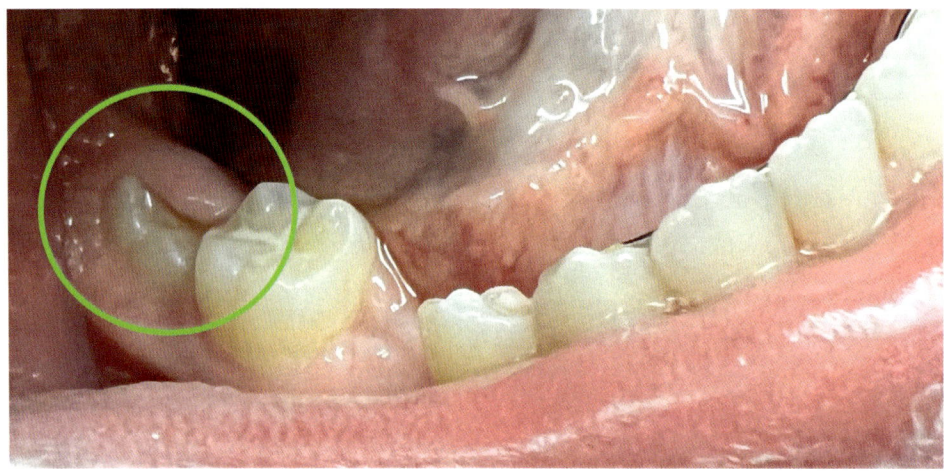

An operculum is a flap of gum tissue partially covering a back molar.

There are several treatment recommendations to alleviate the discomfort caused by an operculum. Over-the-counter pain medications like acetaminophen or ibuprofen can provide temporary relief. A soft diet that doesn't require much chewing can minimize the discomfort from biting into the tissue. Try yogurt, soup, mashed potatoes, or noodles while the operculum is still present. It's also beneficial to clean under the flap and rinse with salt water or alcohol-free mouthwash. For severe cases, such as those of intense pain or signs of infection, contact your dentist. They can assist in cleaning under the flap or performing a minor procedure known as an *operculectomy* to surgically remove it.

What changes to the oral hygiene regimen should happen in this age group?

The basics remain the same—brushing twice daily for two-minutes using a pea-sized amount of toothpaste with fluoride. At this stage, it is expected that most of your child's teeth should be touching side-by-side and so flossing is now required and should be done at least once daily, preferably at bedtime.

Can my child brush on their own or should I still supervise and do it for them?

A good rule of thumb is that once your child has mastered the coordination and fine motor skills necessary to tie their shoelaces, they can then be reasonably expected to brush their own teeth. This doesn't mean you can stop paying attention though. You should still remain involved, ensuring they are doing a good job, monitoring their routine and time spent brushing. If needed, offer guidance and assistance to maintain optimal oral hygiene.

My child struggles with flossing, what can I do to help?

The traditional technique, which involves wrapping floss around the fingers and maneuvering it between the teeth, may still be challenging for your child at this stage. Even some adults struggle with it from time to time! So, aside from flossing your child's teeth for them, you can also try using *flossers*, which are small disposable plastic devices in which a tight piece of floss is suspended from the end of a rigid handle. The handle helps give children more control when moving the floss between the teeth. Whether using these flossers or doing it the old-fashioned way, the floss should be inserted between each tooth and gently brought down just below the gum line. Note that you should be flossing on both sides of each tooth.

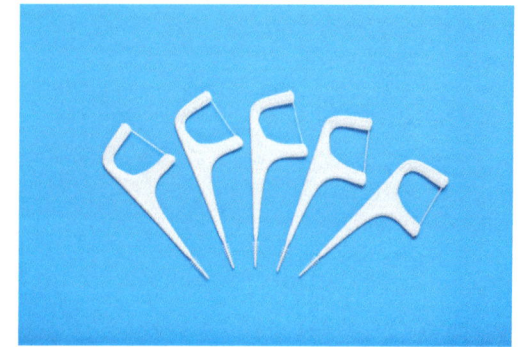

An example of dental flossers.

What are sealants and how do they work?

A dental *sealant* is a resin-based material that is professionally applied to the chewing surfaces of the permanent molars. These surfaces have many narrow *pits and grooves* that are an ideal place for bacteria to make their homes. Here bacteria are sheltered from toothbrush bristles that are too big to penetrate all the way into their depths. Sealant placement is a relatively quick and easy procedure. A dentist paints the viscous resin on the tooth surface, which then hardens within the grooves when exposed to a special light. This forms a protective shield that literally seals up these crevices, thereby blocking small food and bacteria from entering. The overall effect is to produce a more cleansable surface with less risk of decay.

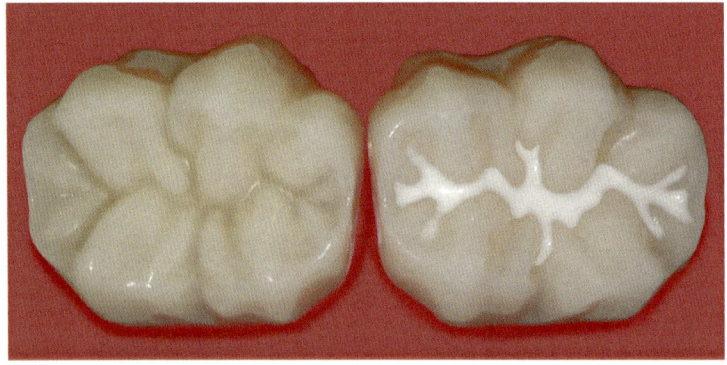

A comparison of molars showing the benefit of sealants.
The molar on the left does not have a sealant, while the one on the right side does.

Are sealants safe and effective?

One of the nice things about dental sealants is that they are *non-invasive*. The procedure is topical and painless, usually not requiring anesthesia or drilling to place them properly. Your child will be able to resume eating right after the procedure is done. Sealants have been used since the 1960s and have only improved in their material composition and effectiveness since that time. They have become not only easier for dentists to work with, but they also provide more durability for the patient. With proper care and monitoring from your dentist, these sealants can last for years. Some research studies have shown that school-aged children with sealants experience three times fewer cavities as compared to children without sealants.[31,32]

I've heard people talk about Bisphenol A (BPA) and sealants. Should I be concerned?

Bisphenol A is a resin commonly found in many different kinds of plastics. It is a concern because there are links between BPA exposure and adverse health effects.[33] While current dental sealants in the United States almost never contain BPA, certain components of the sealant may react with saliva and produce trace amounts of this chemical.[34,35] Thankfully these levels are so low that they would be over a million times smaller than the limits set by the Environmental Protection Agency (EPA) for an average six-year-old.[36] As a result, contemporary sealants should be considered extremely safe.

If sealants are so protective, why not put them on all the teeth?

It's a nice thought, but there are some limitations to what sealants can do. Sealing your child's first permanent molars around six- to seven-years of age hits the sweet spot in a cost-benefit analysis where we would expect to see the greatest return on your investment. In other words, if you're going to pay for a sealant, you want to get the most "bang for your buck." Permanent molars will typically see the highest benefit due not only to their previously mentioned chewing anatomy, the pits and grooves, but also their location in the back of the mouth where children are going to struggle the most to keep them clean. Our other tooth surfaces, like those found on front teeth, are relatively smooth in comparison. Try running your tongue against your front teeth and comparing the feeling to that of the chewing surfaces on your back molars...big difference right? These smooth surfaces do not provide the sealant with anything to latch on to, and so the forces from chewing and daily function would knock them off. While baby molars may also benefit from sealants if they are at high-risk, these molars tend to have wider and shallower grooves, which make them less susceptible compared to their permanent molar counterparts. For all these reasons, we typically think of permanent first molars as being the ideal candidate for dental sealants.

Do sealants have to be done now? Or can we wait until my child is older?

Ultimately, there is no wrong age to get a sealant. If your child is still uncooperative at the dentist, sealants can be deferred until they get a little bit older. It's often better to wait for your child's behavior to improve in the dental chair, rather than try and force an elective procedure on them if they cannot tolerate it. However, a key concept in the placement of sealants is the understanding and estimation of risk. Teeth are at risk as soon as they come into the mouth, and the longer you wait, the greater the chance these teeth may get cavities. Dentists should consider the big picture when making a decision if and when sealants are right for your child.

Should there be any changes to my child's fluoride regimen at this age?

It is still recommended that your child receives professionally applied fluoride therapies at their routine dental visits every six-months. Additionally, for those children deemed to be at high-risk who are not getting adequate fluoride exposure from their home water supply and/or dietary sources, your dentist may elect to increase their supplementation dosage to as much as one-milligram per day.

Now that my child is getting a little older, are there any benefits to using mouthwash?

As discussed in our previous chapter, mouthwashes (rinses) are never a substitute for brushing and flossing. However, in this age group, there may be some very specific indications for why rinsing could be beneficial for your child. These reasons might include providing additional topical fluoride, to treat bacterial infections, to promote good gum health, or combat bad breath. Speak with your dentist to determine whether there is a need and what product will best meet that need. Regardless of what mouthwash is used, the product should be stored in a safe place such that your child will not be able to accidentally consume it inappropriately.

I hear my child grinding their teeth at night, should I be concerned?

Grinding of teeth, also known as *bruxism*, is a fairly common occurrence during one's childhood years, particularly when new teeth are erupting.[37,38] Usually, grinding happens at nighttime, and often children are unaware of it themselves. Instead, it's typically the parents who hear the sounds of the grinding coming from their children's rooms at night. It's unclear why so many children grind their teeth, but some possible explanations include a shifting and inconsistent dental alignment as teeth erupt, stress or nervousness, hyperactivity disorders (like ADHD), and it being a side effect of some medications.[39,40] Signs of grinding can include jaw and facial muscle soreness (particularly when waking in the morning), headaches, small chipping of the front teeth, flattening or wearing down of back teeth, and pain when chewing. Generally though, unless severe, grinding in young children is self-limiting—that is to say, it produces little to no lasting effect and typically goes away on its own.

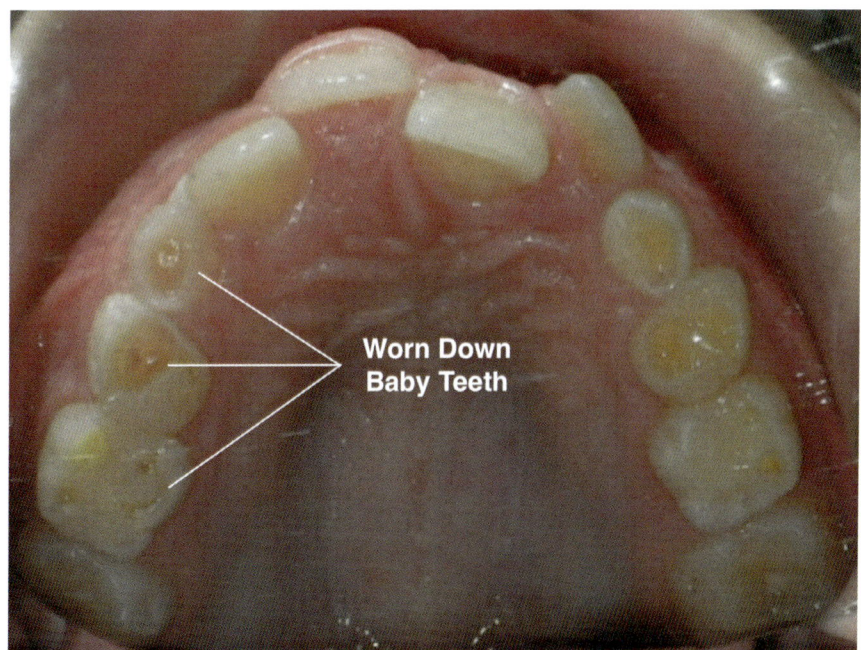

Picture of a seven-year-old's upper teeth.
Note the significant wear seen on the baby teeth, most likely due to severe grinding.

What can I do to help with my child's grinding habits?

The majority of children outgrow the issue with age, but for others it may persist into early adulthood. It is important to try and identify a primary cause for the grinding. Is it related to something anatomic or is it attributable to something psychological? Stress or anxiety-related grinding can be more difficult to address, as it may indicate problems at home or in school. Consider recent lifestyle changes and ask yourself the following questions. Are they overwhelmed and struggling to adapt to the elementary school environment or to their new teachers? Are there problems with bullying? Do they seem hyperactive all throughout the day? The treatment for these situations will involve more than just a simple trip to the dentist. Sometimes a visit to other healthcare professionals and counselors may be indicated.

What about night guards for grinding?

Most children will not need a night guard, as the condition will typically resolve on its own with limited to no damage. However, for those rarer instances involving significant wear or damage to the adult teeth, a night guard may be an appropriate option to help control the effects of your child's bruxism. A night guard can buffer the teeth from damage and provide a flat surface that prevents them from pushing one another into an unstable alignment. These guards are not without their problems in this age group though. First, children must be willing to wear it routinely—this is no small order. Second, when the guard is made, the fit is based on the existing position of your child's teeth. But, in six-months to a year, the guard may no longer fit when new teeth come in and others are lost. Lastly, if made improperly or without attention to detail, the night guard can have lasting negative effects on the bite. We highly recommend having a night guard made by a dentist or orthodontist, rather than purchasing a do-it-yourself type.

Is laser dentistry an option for my child?

Lasers have proven to be a viable option in treating tooth decay and gum issues. Instead of mechanically contacting the tooth with a drill, a laser uses a specific wavelength of light to "cut" through tooth and bone. This removes the vibrations and sounds of the drill that may frighten certain children. Some of the other benefits of lasers include shortened procedure times, cauterization, and a reduced need for local anesthetics (i.e., your child may not need injections to numb their teeth prior to having work done). However, it's important to note that lasers aren't perfect. The cutting action of a laser is accomplished by little micro explosions, and there may be a need to refine the tooth surfaces with a traditional dental drill even after the laser is used. Some procedures may also still require the use of anesthesia depending on how deep the initial cavity is. With that said, depending on the situation and needs, laser dentistry may be an appropriate alternative to consider.

What does it mean if my child's first permanent molar is "stuck"?

Sometimes, as first permanent molars (the six-year molars) make their way into the mouth, they get "caught" on the adjacent baby teeth. This is known as an *ectopic molar,* and the degree of seriousness is dependent on the extent to which the tooth is stuck and the age of the child. On certain occasions, one may be able to see the ectopic molar tipped in the mouth, but sometimes the first molar is visible only on an X-ray. In the accompanying photo, you can see that the lower first molar is trying to come into the mouth, but is being blocked by the baby tooth in front of it.

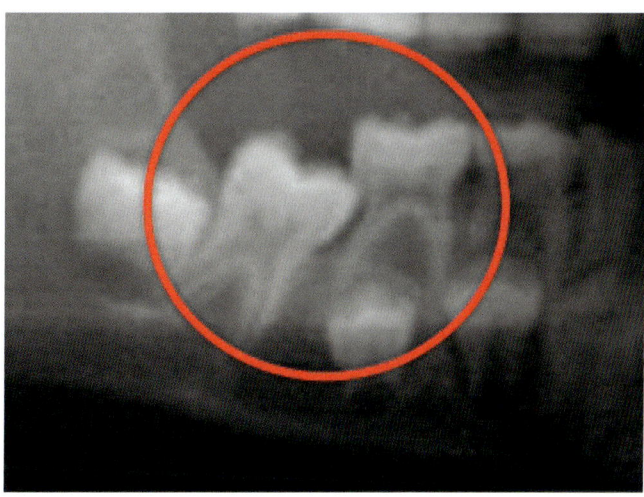

X-ray of lower right first molar that is unable to come in properly due to its angulation.

Treatment is mostly based on how poor the position of the molar is. In mild cases, the problem may fix itself. As the position worsens, a few types of treatments may be required. These include, but are not limited to, extraction of the baby tooth, a partial set of braces, brass springs, or a Halterman appliance.

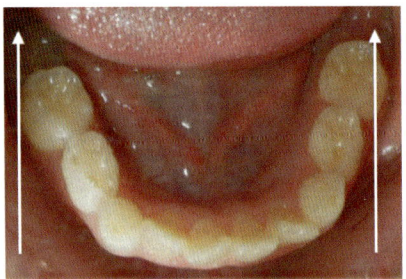
First Molars unable to come in on their own

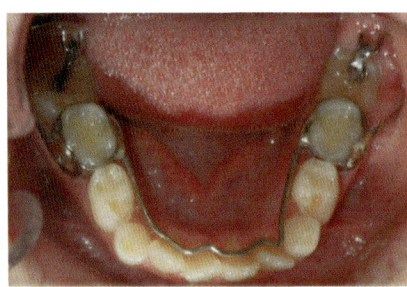
Halterman Appliance

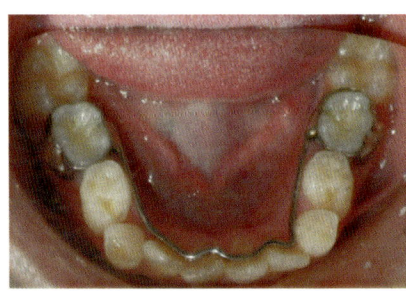
First Molars in proper position

Both lower first molars are ectopic and unable to erupt on their own.
A Halterman appliance is placed to help move the teeth backward to allow them to come in properly.

How long after a baby tooth falls out does it take for the adult tooth come in?

If the baby tooth falls out naturally, it is typically expected for an adult tooth to come in within three-months. However, if the baby tooth was lost early due to trauma, or a large cavity, it may take considerably more time for the adult tooth to erupt in its place. If the adult tooth still fails to make its appearance well beyond the expected eruption date, it is prudent to consult your dentist.

Let's consider an example of a central incisor that did not want to come in when it was supposed to. In this particular case, a boy was first seen at the orthodontist's office at the age of eight-years and two-months, approximately eighteen-months after he had lost his front baby tooth. His parents were worried because his adult tooth had not yet come in, while other teeth around it did. X-rays revealed that the tooth was stuck on the root of the adjacent tooth.

To address the issue, an orthodontic expander was used to widen the dental arch and create more space for the tooth to erupt. Within a year, the tooth in question had normalized well. This highlights the importance of timely dental evaluation and intervention when adult teeth do not erupt within the expected time frame.

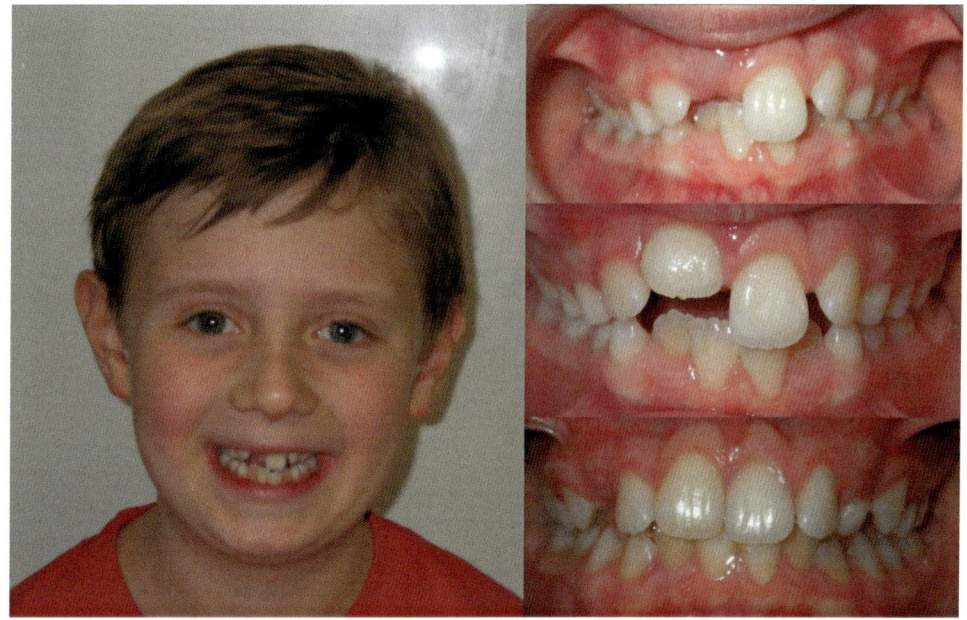

Creating space for an eight-year-old boy's central incisor to erupt.

How concerned should I be if my child chips a permanent front tooth?

Concern should be based on the extent of injury. A mild chip to an adult tooth can have minimal long-lasting effects and can be repaired predictably with an esthetic bonding. Small chips are not considered dental emergencies and treatment can be deferred until your dentist's next available appointment. A large chip (as pictured) likely will be more involved and may even require a root canal and/or a crown. A good rule of thumb is to check if the inner tooth layers are exposed. Under these circumstances, it is best for you to contact your child's dentist sooner rather than later.

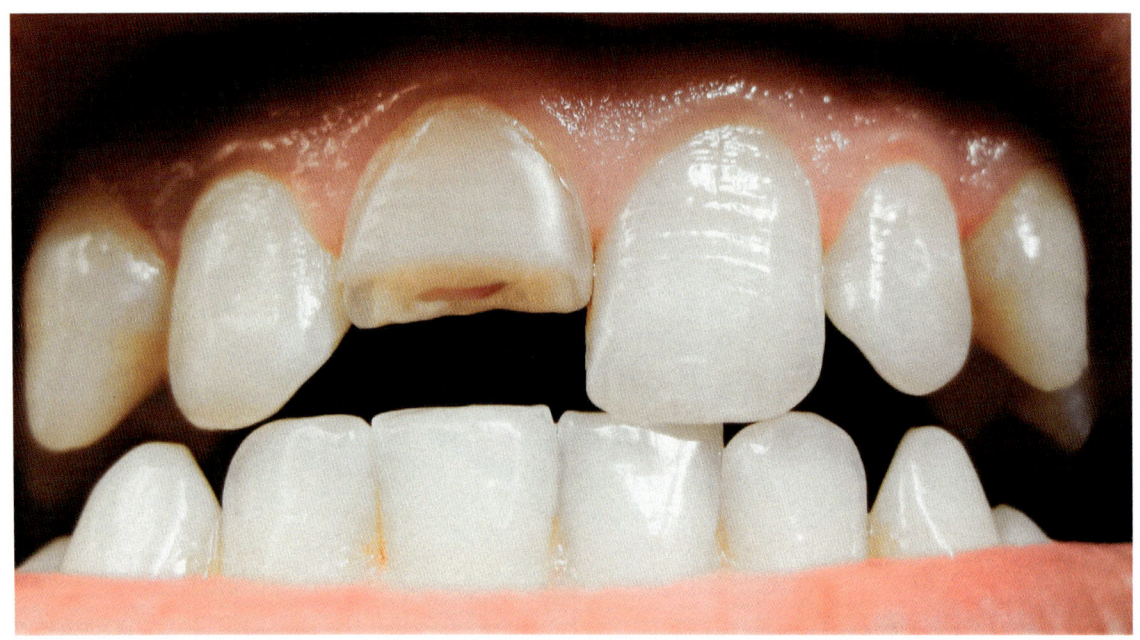

A large chip in a front adult tooth. If you can see a portion of a tooth that is a different color than the outer enamel, it is more serious.

How do I manage a tooth that has been knocked-out?

Treatment depends on whether the tooth knocked-out is an adult or baby tooth. If you are witness to the injury, attempt to recover the tooth and store it in *milk*. Time is of the essence, as the longer the tooth spends out of the mouth, the worse the prognosis! Visit a dentist or emergency department as soon as possible. If you are certain the knocked-out tooth was a permanent tooth, you can re-implant it into its socket yourself. Ensure the tooth is clean before re-implanting it; if it is visibly dirty, you should gently rinse the tooth by running it under a light stream of milk or saline, but do not scrub the tooth or root.[41] Check the tooth's orientation, and once back into the socket, have your child bite down on gauze, wadded-up napkins, or a washcloth to keep it stable while you transport your child to receive follow-up care. If you are unsure if the tooth is permanent or feel uncomfortable re-implanting it yourself, you should bring your child immediately to the dentist or emergency room depending on the extent of the injury and availability of these parties. The re-implanted tooth will need to be splinted with a wire to stabilize the tooth for a few weeks until its mobility decreases. Extensive follow-up and additional treatment are inevitable in these scenarios.

What if I do not have milk readily available to store the tooth?

Storage options ranked best to worst include milk; "Save-a-Tooth" or "Hank's Balanced Salt Solution" products (available in some first aid kits); saliva of the patient (after gently spitting or drooling into a container); saline; or as a last resort—water.[42] It should be emphasized that storing the tooth in any neutral pH liquid is better than keeping it dry. By the way, most of the studies on storing teeth are based on cow's milk...but if you only have almond or oat milk at home, we'd recommend using what you have.

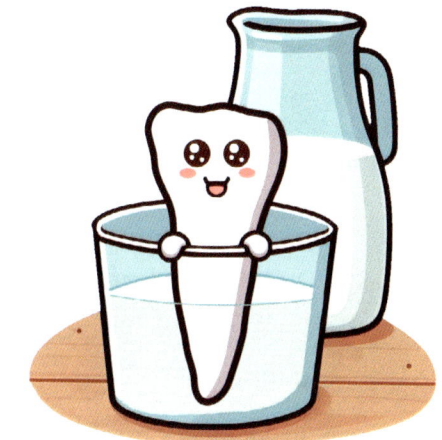

What is the prognosis of a knocked-out tooth at this age?

At this stage in your child's dental development, the adult front teeth that have recently come into the mouth are still considered to be immature. Recall from Chapter 2, that it will take an additional few years for a tooth's root to fully form after it has erupted. These incompletely formed roots may make the teeth more susceptible to being knocked-out, but at the same time, they provide a better capacity for healing than fully mature teeth would have. Therefore, if the tooth is stored properly and brought quickly to the dentist, you have a good chance of saving the tooth. A traumatized tooth will always require additional follow-up in the future, as it can take time to really appreciate the extent of the damage.

"There is nothing permanent except change."

– Heraclitus

Life is never stagnant and neither are our smiles. We hope that the information provided in this chapter has made you feel more prepared to face the inevitable changes coming your way during your child's early school-age years. Embrace the future, be proactive, and remain observant. You will find that the more invested you are in your child's oral health, the greater the return.

CHAPTER 6
AGE EIGHT TO TEN – AN INCISOR INTERMISSION

Where there was once a steady stream of dental changes coming your way, there is now a momentary break in the action. Children of this age are firmly in the *mixed dentition*, an in-between phase, with a mixture of both baby and adult teeth present. Your child's development is also in an in-between phase of sorts. They are no longer dependent on you for everything, but not yet fully self-sufficient. While the dental aspects of this stage may seem relatively stable, it's important to recognize that much growth is still happening in a child's life. Social and cognitive development are in full swing and they are embracing new experiences and challenges. This stage is characterized by increased engagement in sports and hobbies, forming new relationships, and perhaps even learning to appreciate other's perspectives. Whether it's grinning after a big game or trying to captivate someone special with their charm, they're going to need their smiles by their side.

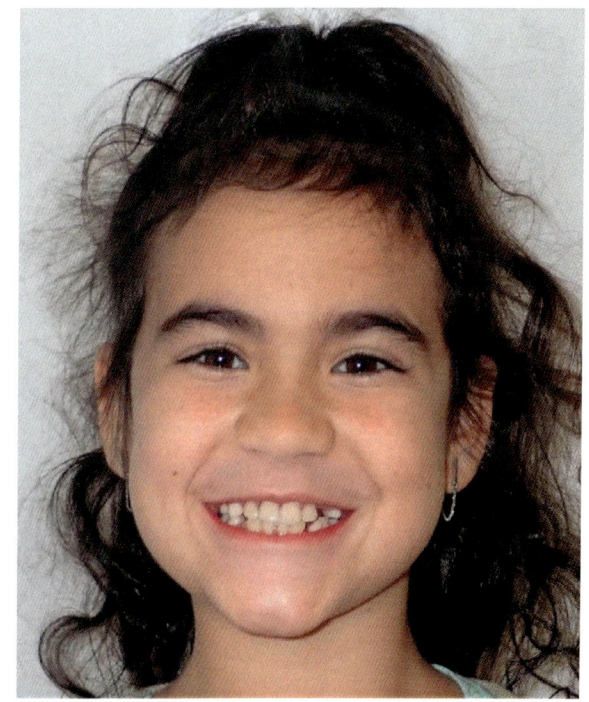

Smiling photo of a nine-year-old.
Note that all the incisors are in their position and no major changes are occurring outside the gums.

What, if anything, is happening with the teeth at this age?

We like to call this period "intermission" because there is a short pause from the process of baby teeth falling out and being replaced by permanent teeth. In a sense, the teeth are in a period of *stability*. Though we do not see any changes occurring in the mouth, much is still happening underneath the gums and in the bone. The canines and premolars are now developing, getting larger, and gradually breaking down the roots of the baby teeth that they will replace. During this time, it is crucial to pay extra attention to their position and angulation.

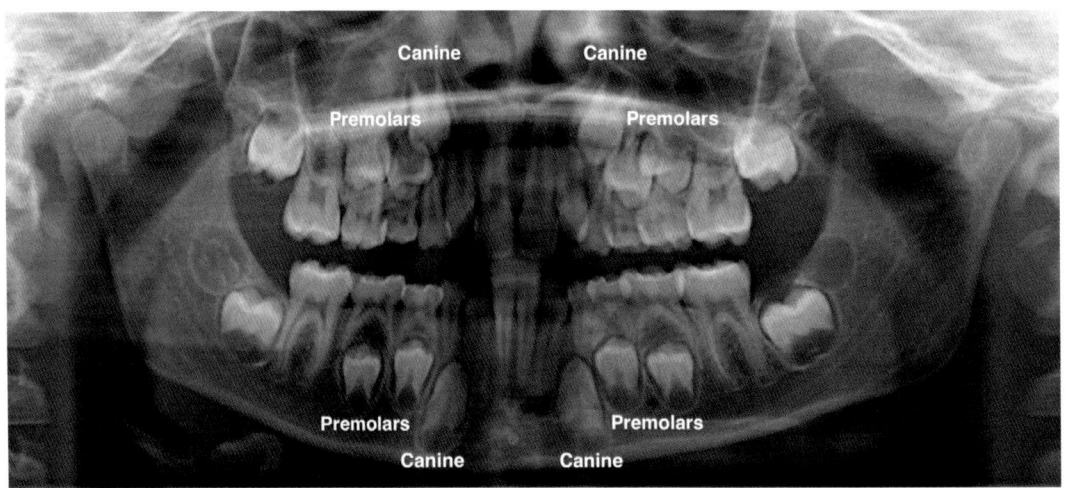

X-ray at age eight. Note the developing adult teeth.

What is an "impacted" canine?

Puppies can be mischievous scamps. Canine teeth can do silly things too, and may develop and migrate in a different direction than we would like. This may lead to an *impacted tooth*, which is a tooth that is stuck or blocked from coming in properly. While this can happen to any tooth, from an orthodontic perspective, it is the impaction of the canines that is of considerable importance. Prevention of an impacted tooth is one of the reasons that early interceptive orthodontic treatment might be indicated for your child. Note the position of the upper canines in the earlier of the two following X-rays. While not perfect, they are reasonably positioned with a vertical angulation, and a decision to monitor them was made. Now look at the X-ray at age eleven. You can see that their position has worsened and there is now overlap with the adjacent teeth. In some instances, extractions of baby teeth to create space for the impacted tooth may provide a path for eruption and prevent further more invasive treatments. However, in other instances, this early intervention is not enough, and teeth may need additional help to be brought into the dental arch. This advanced intervention may involve the use of surgeries in which the teeth are physically guided into the mouth with chains and braces.

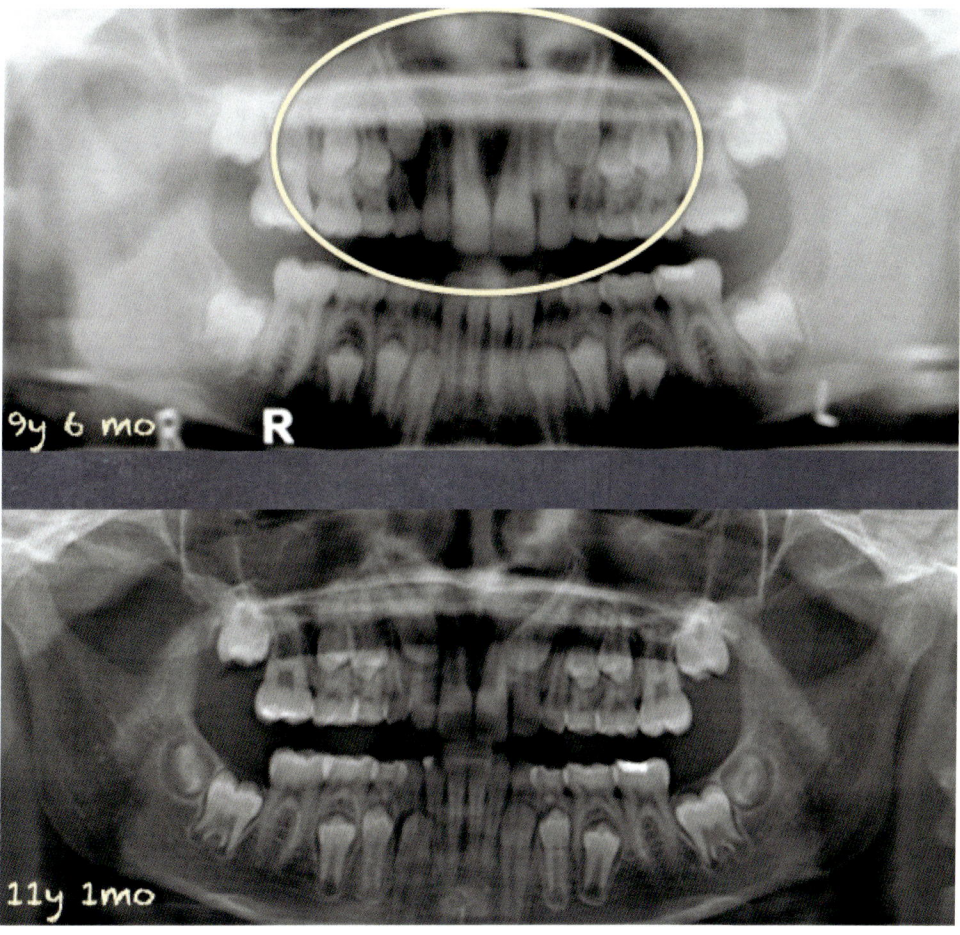

Note the changes in the upper permanent canines. At age nine, they were in a reasonable position. However, a year and a half later, they have turned inwards and now are overlapping other permanent teeth.

Should there be any changes to the oral hygiene routine?

Your child should now feel very comfortable brushing and flossing on their own. How good of a job are they doing? That's the million-dollar question. The dentist and hygienist will certainly let you know at their cleaning appointments, but don't be afraid to look in their mouth and ask them to re-brush or floss when necessary. The earlier your child builds a consistent routine, the better.

What is gingivitis?

Gingivitis is a condition characterized by inflammation of the gums that surround and support the teeth. It is primarily caused by the presence of bacteria and the body's response against it. These bacteria are tiny organisms that can normally only be seen under a microscope. In the absence of good oral hygiene practices, these bacteria can accumulate in such high numbers that they can be seen with the naked-eye, forming a sticky film over the teeth known as *dental plaque*. This plaque is most commonly found right along the gum line, but with gross negligence of oral hygiene, it may cover the whole tooth. Just as the bacterial products from plaque promote the formation of cavities on the teeth, so too can they negatively affect the gums. Inflammation from gingivitis turns the gums from a healthy pink to a red, irritated, swollen structure. Though gingivitis is commonly seen in this age group, it is something that we battle against throughout life. For more information on gingivitis and its progression to the more severe form of the disease known as periodontitis, refer to Chapter 11.

My child has bad breath. What is causing this?

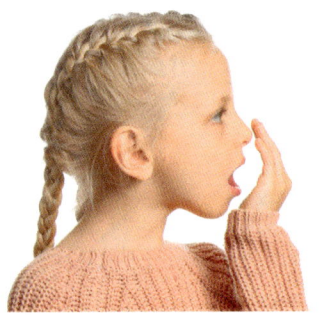

Bad breath, also known as *halitosis*, may be a troublesome condition for both parents and young children, as it can be quite socially embarrassing and unpleasant to be around. There are a number of possible causes for this condition in children, including diet, poor oral hygiene, or childhood illnesses such as gastroesophageal reflux disease (GERD).[43]

Dietary choices are a common cause of bad breath. Certain foods that adults know all too well, such as garlic and onion, can lead to a lingering odor in the mouth. Perhaps more importantly, the consumption of sugary drinks and snacks in combination with poor oral hygiene contributes to the growth of bacteria that leads to malodorous breath. If your child is aware of the problem, it is a great time to review the importance of flossing and brushing regularly.

Sometimes the odor may still be present even when oral hygiene appears impeccable. Consider a respiratory infection that leads to a post-nasal drip or gastric reflux causing stomach acids to flow up into the mouth. Both of these conditions can lead to halitosis and a bad taste in the mouth. Children who are mouth breathers, including those whose nasal passages are obstructed, are also more prone to having bad breath. Mouth breathing dries out the oral environment and causes odors in the mouth to be more prominent.[44] By noticing and addressing halitosis, you may be helping your child not only to have fresh breath and good oral hygiene, but also improving their overall health.

What can I do to combat my child's bad breath?

Identifying the causes of bad breath will be the most important step in addressing it. Ensure your child is following proper oral hygiene, including brushing their tongue to remove odor-causing bacteria that may be hiding in its furrows. Alcohol-free mouth rinses may also be helpful in controlling bad breath at this age. If your child's mouth seems dry, have them take frequent sips of water throughout the day or use sugar-free lozenges, gums, or sucking candies to encourage more saliva to flow. If the child is experiencing other issues like heartburn, speak with your pediatrician to assess for systemic causes of bad breath such as medical conditions, hormonal imbalances, and side effects of certain medications.

What is Phase 1 Orthodontic Treatment?

Phase 1 treatment is a first round of orthodontic care done at an earlier age than traditional braces. It is common to start Phase 1 treatment in the eight- to ten-year-old age group, as the aforementioned *stability* of the teeth during this time makes it convenient for early interceptive procedures. Phase 1 therapy aims to decrease the complexity and scope of a second, more comprehensive, round of orthodontics that will usually take place in early to late adolescence. While we will delve into more details about comprehensive orthodontics in Chapter 9, for now, let us consider some of the early bite issues that parents should be on the lookout for.

Anterior Crossbite

An *anterior crossbite* means one or more of the lower incisors are in front of the upper incisors; the reverse of the normal relationship. This can be a result of the way the teeth erupted, or it may be a result of a jaw disharmony. Treatment to correct this issue ranges from simply applying pressure to the teeth with a tongue depressor, to the use of removable appliances or a partial set of braces, all the way up to a type of special headgear. As with most conditions, the sooner the problem is identified, the easier treatment tends to be.

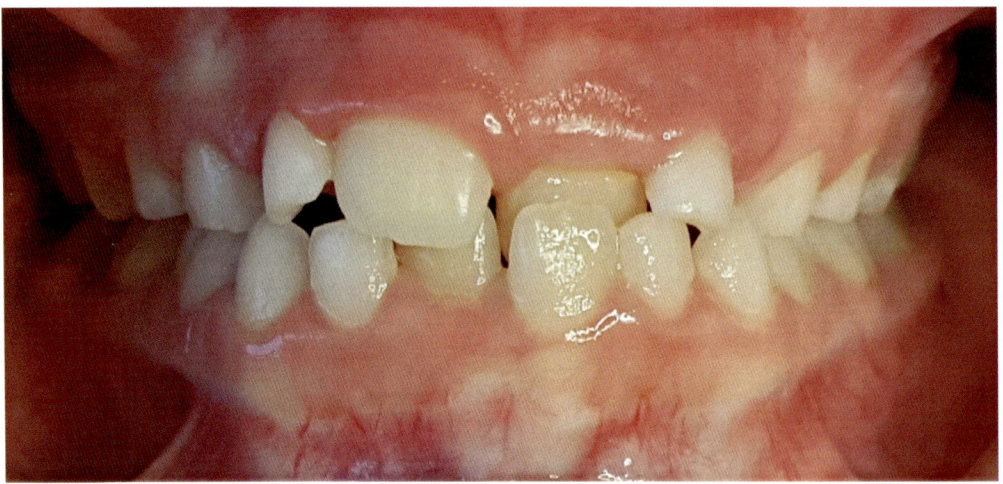

Anterior Crossbite. All upper teeth should be overlapping the lower teeth.

Posterior Crossbite

A *posterior crossbite* occurs when the back teeth do not overlap properly in the lateral (side-to-side) direction. This can occur with only one of the back teeth, one full side (right or left), or both sides simultaneously. The posterior crossbite can result from either a dental or a skeletal disharmony, or on occasion, it might be related to both. If the crossbite is of dental origin, sometimes it may not be immediately treated at a young age and will instead be combined with braces later on. If a crossbite is of skeletal origin (because of a narrow upper jaw), a special appliance known as an *expander* is used to correct the problem. See Chapter 9 for more information regarding expanders and crossbites. In the picture below, note the difference between the overlap of the back teeth on the right side versus the left side.

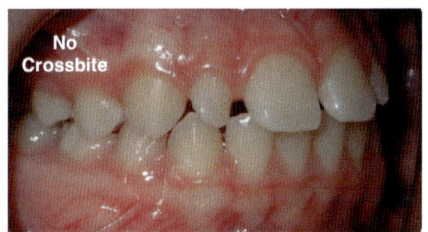 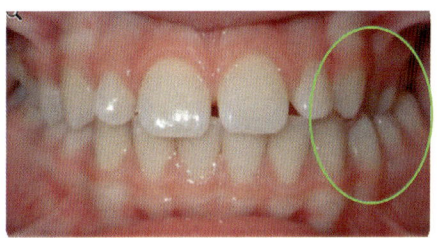 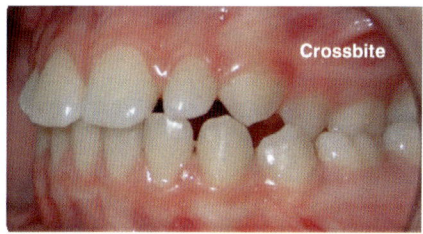

Note that on the patient's left side (right side of the picture), the top teeth do not overlap the bottom teeth properly.

Thumb Sucking

We are now at the age in which thumb sucking habits are likely to cause lasting permanent effects, such as pushing the front teeth out, narrowing the upper jaw, and affecting growth patterns. The eight-year-old girl's teeth pictured below shows that her upper incisors are tilted forward and the lower incisors are tilted back. The distance created between them is almost ten-millimeters, which is significantly higher than normal. Also, note the narrowed palate that has resulted from her thumb placement on the roof of her mouth. If your child is still sucking their thumb at this age, it is critical to get help to eliminate this habit before it's too late.

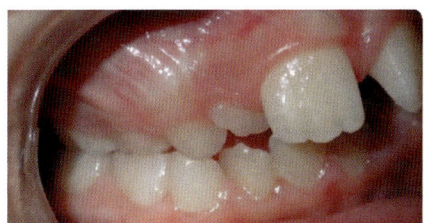 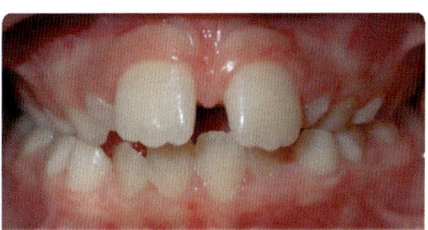 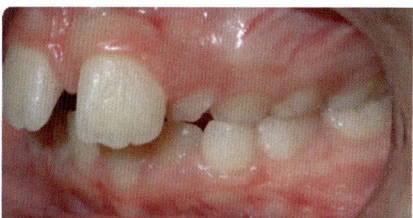

Thumb sucking typically leads to the upper front teeth pushing out, lower front teeth tipping back, and can negatively affect jaw growth.

Mouth Breathing

Similar to thumb sucking, mouth breathing and snoring can also have long-lasting effects on the development of your child's bite and jaws. Kids should be able to comfortably breathe through their nose, especially when they sleep. Mouth breathing tends to dry out the mouth, which does not allow saliva to work to its fullest extent to help protect against cavities. Another negative effect of mouth breathing is the change in position of the lower jaw. Mouth breathing forces the jaw open for a greater portion of the day. This causes the jaw to grow downward instead of forward, creating an open-bite (a vertical gap between the front teeth). An increase in open-bite usually allows the tongue to thrust forward into this space, making the open-bite worse in a vicious cycle. Treatment for mouth breathing may include expansion (making the upper jaw wider) with the intent of improving airway volume, and often a dentist may recommend a visit to the ear, nose, and throat (ENT) doctor. An ENT can evaluate the adenoids and tonsils which may also impair breathing. The adenoids and tonsils are discussed in greater detail in Chapter 12.

Severe Crowding (Crooked Teeth)

Crowding occurs when two or more teeth are vying for the same limited space in the mouth, causing misalignment and overlap. Severe crowding at this age is often an ominous sign of what is to come, as the problem almost never corrects itself and will likely get worse with time. In some instances, crowding may be treated by expansion at this age. In other cases, strategic extractions of baby teeth may be indicated to create space. If there is significant crowding at an early age, it is definitely a good idea to seek an orthodontist for their opinion.

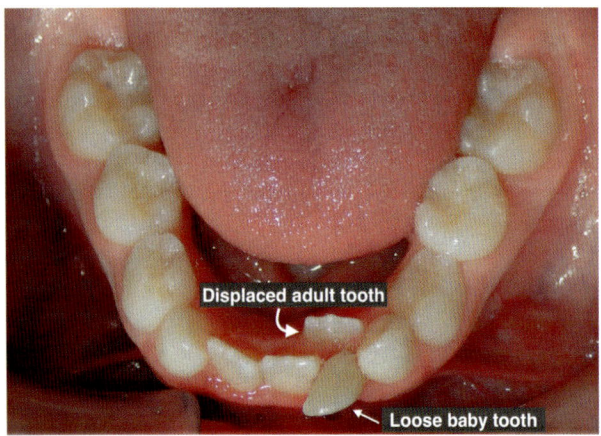

Severe crowding seen in the lower teeth. In this example, only three of the four adult lower incisors are visible, with no room for the fourth incisor to erupt. There is a large difference in the amount of space present compared to the amount of space needed, and so, the fourth incisor does not have any place to erupt.

Front Teeth Jutting Out

"Bunny teeth" are common in this age group. It's a term used to describe when the upper front teeth stick out further than their lower counterparts. Though it may appear that the fault lies squarely with the position of the upper incisors, the gap may actually be due to a small lower jaw. If the lower jaw is too small relative to the upper jaw, the horizontal distance between the teeth will be increased. It is important to discern the true cause of the discrepancy. Once this is determined, a proper treatment plan can be created. This specific issue is often misdiagnosed.

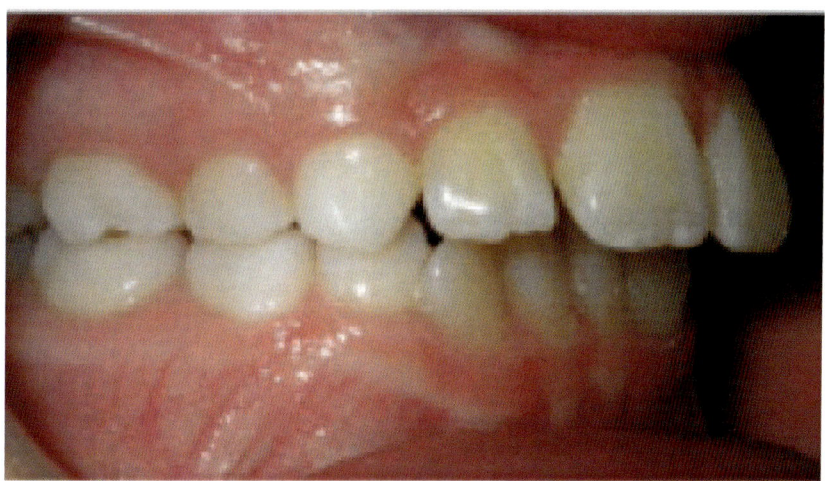

Bunny teeth are upper incisors that stick relatively too far out.

Speech Problems

Speech is a combination of breath, vocal cords, tongue, jaw, and tooth position. Changes to any of these may have an effect on the way words sound. Often, speech issues are picked up at the elementary school level. Speech-language pathologists (SLPs) can play a vital role in improving your child's speech, which can have many positive effects. The SLP's goal is to help the child speak more clearly given their existing anatomy. Open-bites and large overjet (where the upper incisors protrude significantly far ahead of their lower counterparts) are two types of anatomical issues that can cause speech problems. Improving these issues will also allow for speech correction to occur more easily.

"Appearances are often deceiving."
- Aesop

Despite the relative tranquility of this period, there are critical events happening just beyond our view. Be careful not to get lulled into a false sense of security. That goes for check-ups too—just because your child may have had a recent dentist visit with "no cavities" doesn't mean that everything is sunshine and roses. Your child's oral health isn't solely their teeth. It's time to start paying more attention to the gums and developing bite. This is a great time to consider an orthodontic evaluation if you haven't already done so. We hope you've enjoyed this brief intermission; the next chapter in your child's smile story is about to begin!

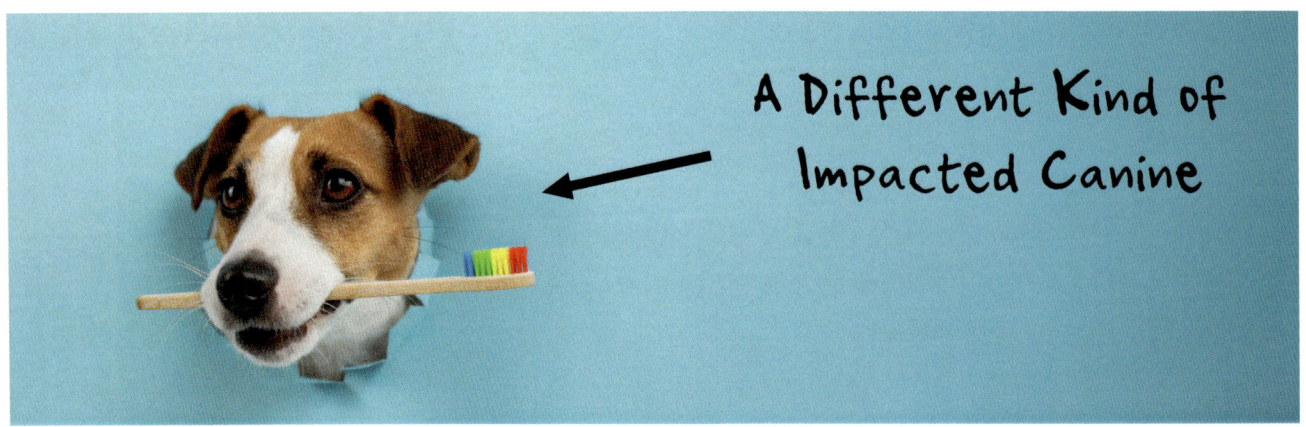

A Different Kind of Impacted Canine

CHAPTER 7
AGE TEN TO TWELVE – TWEEN TOOTH TELL-ALLS

Let's try to savor our children being "precious little ones" for just a bit longer—for puberty is right around the corner and before long you may not even recognize the person they'll become. Middle school is on the horizon, and it can be a tough go for some children, fraught with social and academic challenges. Peer pressure can weigh heavily on your child during this age, and they may encounter difficult internal conflicts as a result. Their dental development is also at a crossroads with pivotal events influencing its future direction. If all the pieces fall neatly into place, we'll be on the path to success, but just a few missteps, and we may be set on a dangerous track where their smile's development could go off course.

What's happening from a dental perspective at this age?

This is the stage where the twelve remaining baby teeth naturally fall out, and hopefully the adult teeth that replace them come in as expected. The baby canines and molars will be succeeded by the adult canines and premolars. In kids where severe crowding exists, managing the spaces created when baby teeth fall out is of critical importance.

What are space maintainers?

A *space maintainer* is an appliance used to maintain space. Well, duh! What does that really mean? Once again, we must emphasize the importance of specific sequences that teeth follow when they exfoliate and erupt. We would like to think that nature always follows this set order, but sometimes life has other plans for us. In some instances, a baby tooth (or teeth) may need to be extracted years before it was supposed to naturally fall out. This could happen due to a large cavity, infection, or trauma. When a tooth is lost prematurely, the adjacent teeth will sometimes inappropriately slide over into the free space—they can be quite greedy! This creates a problem, because our baby teeth have a job to do, serving as placeholders for the adult teeth. A premature change can block out a developing tooth, can shift a midline, and can negatively affect the bite. This is where space maintainers can come into play. These metal devices are cemented in place and essentially hold back the adjacent teeth to prevent this shifting and space loss. Space maintainers are a relatively simple and cost-effective means of mitigating the effects of early tooth loss.

Space Maintainer – Lower Lingual Holding Arch – This specific space maintainer has two bands (that look like tooth rings) soldered to a connector wire.

If my child is participating in contact sports, should they be wearing a mouthguard?

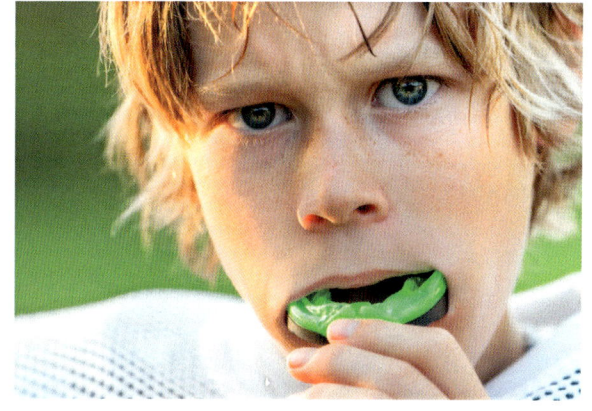

Almost all sports have an inherent risk of injuries due to collisions, falls, and impacts with equipment. The protective and positive results of wearing a mouthguard have been demonstrated in numerous studies and tests.[45] However, the rules regarding mouthguards are inconsistent across towns and athletic organizations. Thus, it becomes crucial for parents and coaches to actively encourage or require children to wear mouthguards and other protective equipment like helmets and facemasks when appropriate. Our recommendation is clear—if there is any possibility of striking the face with a ball, puck, elbow, or head-butt while playing a sport, then your child should be wearing a mouthguard.

What type of mouthguard should I get?

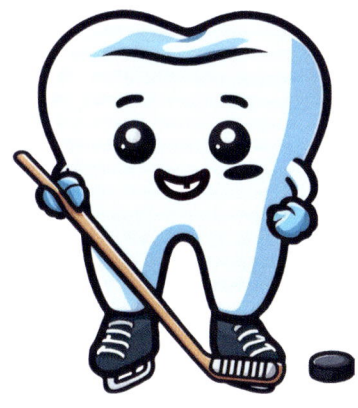

There are three types of commonly available mouthguards, each with its own advantages and disadvantages. *Stock mouthguards* are prefabricated devices that are available in most sporting goods stores—these are the most basic option. While they are generally inexpensive, they offer the least amount of protection and the lowest level of comfort. Your child will inconveniently need to bite down in order to keep the mouthguard in place without falling out. We recommend avoiding these unless there is no other feasible option. *Boil-and-bite* style mouthguards are also available in stores and are relatively inexpensive, but are more customizable. They are heated in boiling water, which allows the mouthguard to be shaped to the child's teeth for a better fit and improved comfort. Lastly, the *custom-made* mouthguard is professionally fabricated by your child's dentist, providing a superior fit with the most comfort and protection. This style is likely to be more expensive than the commercially available alternatives.

Selecting the right mouthguard should also take into account any unique circumstances your child may have. For example, if your child has braces, it is critical that the mouthguard is labeled "for-braces" on the package. A boil-and-bite mouthguard could get stuck in the braces during molding and lead to a very uncomfortable Friday night! Regardless of the mouthguard you choose, injuries can still happen, but by taking the appropriate precautions, you can at least minimize the extent of the damage.

How do I care for their mouthguard?

It is recommended that you or your child clean their mouthguard after each use. Use cool, soapy water to clean all the surfaces before storage. We recommend against using very hot water to make sure that the mouthguard does not deform from the heat. Hopefully, there was no food on the child's teeth prior to wearing the mouthguard, but do not be shy about brushing it with a toothbrush and toothpaste as needed. Ever so often, you should check to ensure it still has a good fit and that there are no significant signs of wear and tear that might necessitate replacement. As children grow and their teeth transition, their mouthguards will need to be replaced periodically. Children should also be discouraged from chewing on their mouthguards while in use. If your child is a basketball fan, they may notice that Steph Curry is constantly chewing on his mouthguard. What they probably don't realize is that as a professional athlete he can afford to get a new one made each game!

My child's gums bleed when they brush or floss. Should I be concerned?

Healthy gums do not bleed! If your child's gums are bleeding while brushing, there is a problem—and that problem is almost certainly gingivitis. In Chapter 6, we defined gingivitis as inflammation of the gums (gingiva) in response to dental plaque around the gum line. Inflamed gums are often red, swollen, and bleed easily. This diseased state can be reversed by improving the quality and consistency of oral hygiene. We often hear from children and parents that the reason they avoid flossing is because it makes their gums bleed. In fact, the only solution to this problem is that they need to floss more! As the flossing routine becomes more consistent, the gums will return to health and the bleeding will gradually subside until it no longer happens at all.

My child still has a space between their two front teeth. Will it close on its own?

This space between your child's incisors is known as a *diastema*, and it is quite common in this age group. As more and more of the adult teeth begin to erupt, the alignment of the incisors may tighten up, reducing or closing this space. In the associated photos, note how the gap closed without any professional intervention. However, sometimes the diastema persists into adulthood, and depending on the size of the gap and your child's esthetic desires, this space can be closed with orthodontic tooth movement or dental restorations. Occasionally, a piece of tissue between the two front teeth called a *labial frenum* is partially responsible for this space. More on this topic in Chapter 11.

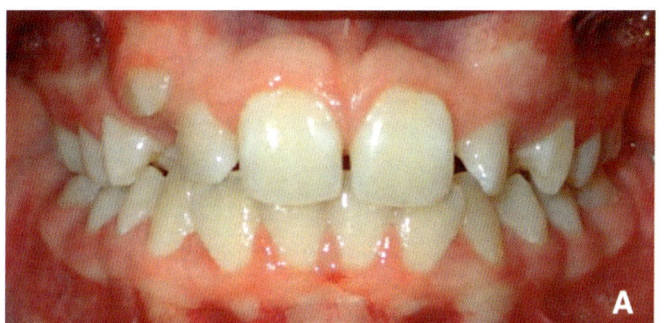 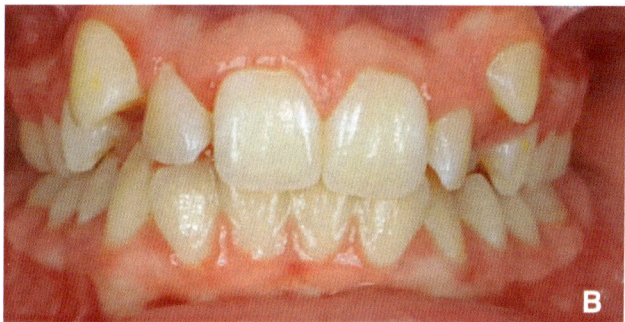

Photos taken eleven-months apart. Note that the canines are just starting to break through the gums. In picture B, the canines are further down, and the space between the two front teeth has become smaller.

My child has frequent canker sores. What can I do to help?

Canker sores, more formally known as *aphthous ulcers*, are essentially breaks in the soft tissue lining of the mouth. They appear as shallow craters with a white, tan, or yellowish center and a bright red border. They may typically be found on the lips, inner cheeks, underneath the tongue, and at the back of the mouth, also known as the soft palate. These sores are considered *idiopathic*, meaning they are a condition that arises spontaneously with no identifiable cause. Canker sores can be considerably painful and interfere with a child's desire to eat. They are non-contagious and not associated with other systemic findings such as fever or swellings. These ulcerations tend to be recurrent, coming back from time to time, but not necessarily in the same spots. They typically begin around adolescence or early childhood and will often continue into adulthood. Estimates vary, but around 20 percent of the general population experience these frustrating ulcers.[46]

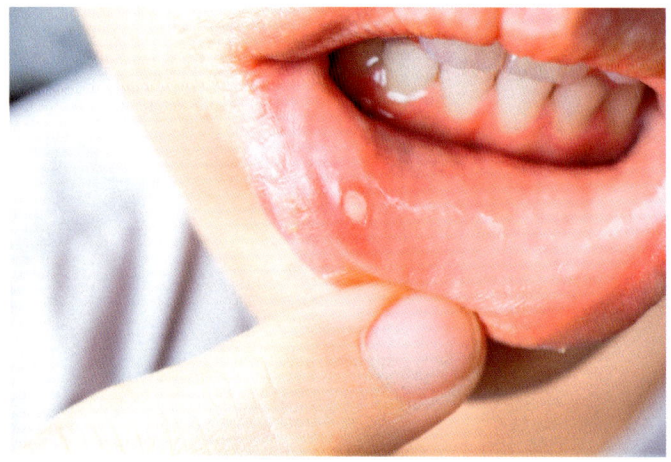

Canker sore on the lower lip.

What can I do to help with my child's canker sores?

Children usually do not require any active treatment for their canker sores. They'll typically heal on their own in approximately one- to two-weeks, although the larger ones may persist for longer periods of time. In general, children suffering from canker sores should avoid spicy or salty foods that may irritate the exposed ulcers. In situations where the ulcers are producing significant pain, such that your child's daily functions are limited, active treatment may be appropriate. Saltwater rinses, while temporarily irritating, may help speed up the healing process. Children should also be encouraged to drink plenty of fluids, especially if they are refusing to eat, to prevent dehydration and encourage healing. Over-the-counter pain medications like Tylenol may be effective in reducing the discomfort they are experiencing. Topical coating agents can also be used to cover the ulcer and prevent food or teeth from rubbing against it. For recurrent cases, dentists may also prescribe various medications, including rinses or gels directed at reducing and controlling inflammation and pain.

Are there any other causes of ulcers in the mouth?

Yes, there are a number of other reasons your child may be developing oral ulcers. Trauma, such as that from an accidental lip, cheek, or tongue bite, can cause an ulcer. Traumatic ulcers may also result from the sharp edges of orthodontic appliances, like brackets, rubbing against the soft tissues of the mouth. Certain viruses common to childhood, including Herpes and Coxsackie, can produce distinctive ulcers as well. Children with certain medical conditions, such as Crohn's disease, are also at an elevated risk of developing ulcerations throughout their GI tract, including the oral cavity.[47] A review of the history, frequency, size, and location of the ulcers with your child's dentist can provide helpful clues as to their root cause.

My child has gastric reflux. How might that affect their teeth?

Gastroesophageal reflux disease (GERD) is a condition in which acidic stomach juices inappropriately back-flow through the digestive tract and potentially rise up into the mouth. These stomach acids are strong and sufficiently powerful to wear and break down teeth. The results of this *erosion* become irreversible over time. Most commonly, it is noted on the biting surfaces of molars and the backside of incisors. As the enamel is dissolved away, a host of negative effects including sensitivity, discoloration, and eventual tooth loss, may occur. Dental erosion can also be the result of poor dietary habits, like sucking lemons, or drinking copious amounts of soda containing citric acid. If your child has GERD, the best course of action would be to consult your pediatrician to receive appropriate treatment to control the underlying condition. It is not recommended to brush the teeth immediately after they are bathed in acid, as they will be in a more vulnerable state, and scrubbing them could further the damage. Instead, one should rinse with water to help neutralize the acids in the mouth.

Why are my child's teeth sensitive to cold things?

Cold sensitivity can be the result of many factors. The most frequent cause is the presence of a cavity that has compromised tooth structure and exposed portions of the tooth that are normally insulated from the oral environment. In some cases, cold sensitivity may be due to other anatomic factors, such as gingival recession, where the gums do not fully cover a tooth's root surface (further discussed in Chapter 11). Previously traumatized teeth are also at an elevated risk for developing cold sensitivity, and this can indicate a worsening prognosis as it relates to nerve damage. When seeking to determine the cause of sensitivity, try to pinpoint if only one tooth, multiple teeth, or perhaps all the teeth are affected. Sometimes pain can radiate to multiple teeth and understanding where the issue is coming from helps to make proper treatment decisions.

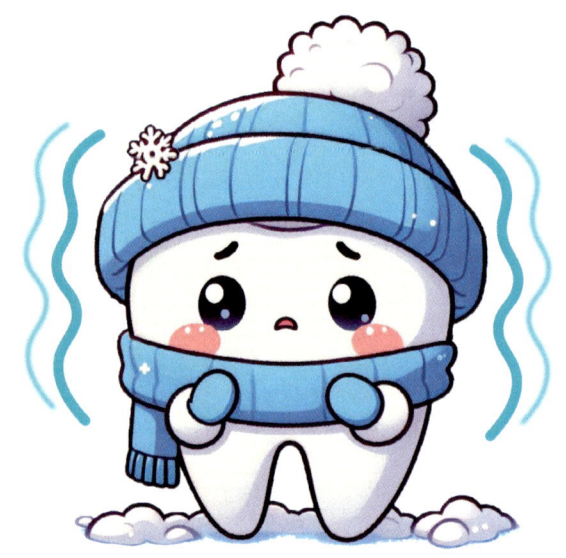

What can be done to combat cold sensitivity?

If you and your child have been following up with routine dental examinations, the probability of the cold sensitivity coming from a very large cavity is quite low. If your child has not had routine dental check-ups, and the issue is indeed a cavity, your child's dentist will review options to remove the decay and restore the tooth. Any changes to previously traumatized teeth, such as a recent discoloration, should be discussed with your dentist so that they may take X-rays to examine for deterioration of the nerve. "But what if the sensitivity is coming from all the teeth?" you may ask. Generalized low-level sensitivity can be treated with special toothpastes, like Sensodyne, that have active ingredients designed to prevent the nerves from firing off pain signals. Look for the ingredient "Potassium Nitrate" on the back of the box.

My child is prone to getting cavities, could they have "soft teeth"?

It is very unlikely that you or your child legitimately have "soft teeth" that would impact their risk of getting cavities. Only rarely—we're talking 1 in 4,000—are children born with genetic conditions like *amelogenesis imperfecta* or *dentinogenesis imperfecta*, which significantly affect the quality and composition of a tooth's structure, making them comparatively "soft."[48] These conditions are generally obvious, as the affected children would have teeth that appear significantly yellow/brown, pitted, and deformed. The term "soft teeth" is usually misused and often said as an excuse that puts the blame for getting cavities on something uncontrollable. In truth, the cause for cavities in the vast majority of cases is always the same—bacteria, sugars, and inadequate hygiene practices. Though certain children may be genetically more susceptible to getting cavities, proper hygiene almost always eliminates those concerns.

Is my pre-teen at risk of getting oral cancer from HPV? Should they get the HPV vaccine?

HPV, the *Human Papilloma Virus*, is associated with a number of different oral lesions. Some strains of the virus simply cause harmless growths that look like oral warts on the lips, cheeks, or gums. Other strains are linked with the devastating development of oral and oropharyngeal (back of the throat) cancers. In fact, approximately 4 percent of all cancers are associated with HPV infection, and they may affect both women and men.[49] Most oral cancers develop in older individuals, particularly among smokers who have put themselves at significant risk throughout their lives, but there has been a recent shift in which more and more young people are being affected by oral cancers linked to HPV. Oral cancer is currently among the ten most common cancers globally, and given that a viable HPV vaccine exists, we support the CDC recommendation that the vaccine be administered to children aged eleven- to twelve-years-old. It can even be given to kids as young as nine.[50, 51] This is an ideal age to get the vaccine, before your child may become sexually active and exposed to the virus.

"All people are the same; only their habits differ."

– Confucius

As your child loses their remaining baby teeth, it is more important than ever to ensure their oral hygiene routines have become an ingrained tradition. Impress upon them that a full set of permanent teeth means that there are no more "do-overs," and from here on out their smile story is written in ink, not pencil. Brushing and flossing are the keys to the kingdom, and an empire built on this habit is a powerful one. Children may often feel invincible when young, but as a parent, you have the maturity to know better. Use your judgment to safeguard them when appropriate. Make wearing a mouthguard as much a part of the game as lacing up their cleats. Get them vaccinated to promote a lifetime of well-being. Their smile is worth protecting.

CHAPTER 8
AGE TWELVE AND BEYOND – PERMANENT PERFECTION

At last, we are at the culmination of your child's smile story—a full complement of adult teeth. As a teenager reaches this age, they find themselves on the cusp of significant physical and emotional change. Puberty begins to influence their growth and development, with females often sprouting taller than their male classmates. By extension, these changes also affect the growth of the jaws, particularly in boys who may develop a prominent "manly" chin. Their attitudes may change too; expect some moodiness and back-talk fueled by a potent mix of hormones and stress. Don't take it personally though…sometimes they just need some space. Despite the challenges of puberty, it remains important to not neglect one's oral health. Whether it's getting braces on, contemplating wisdom teeth removal, or making esthetic improvements to their smile, this chapter delves into the unique dental issues adolescents face during this transformative time in life.

What are the last permanent teeth to come in?

At around twelve-years of age the permanent second molars will erupt all the way in the back of your child's mouth. Similar to when the last set of teeth came in, your child may experience transient teething discomfort or a possible operculum (see Chapter 5 for a refresher). For most children, these molars will complete the set of permanent teeth that they will have room to accommodate in their mouth.

What if my teenager still has baby teeth?

Repeat after me—sequence matters more than timing! We have seen preteens with all their adult teeth in, and older teenagers with multiple baby teeth still present. Nature gives us many variations of normal and everyone's timeline is slightly different. What *is* important is monitoring the order in which teeth come in, and ensuring that there are no problems within the gums or bones that would impede the proper sequence. Dentists and orthodontists will take a *Panoramic X-ray* to ensure everything is proceeding according to plan. Panoramic X-rays ("PANs" for short) are wider images that allow the dentist to visualize all the teeth and their relative positions in one shot. The PAN can also give the dentist a great view of the patient's jawbones to ensure no pathology is present.

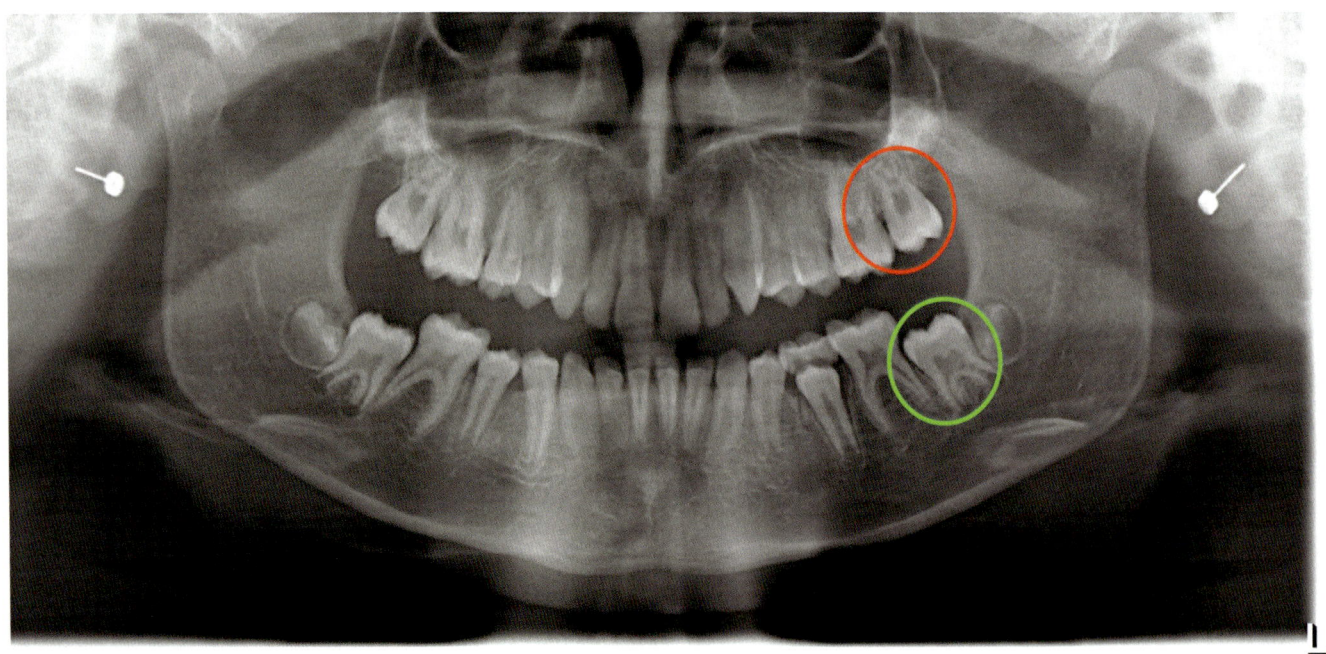

A panoramic X-ray on a twelve-year-old girl. Note that the upper twelve-year molars have erupted into the arch as seen with the red circle, and the lower twelve-year molars, circled in green, will erupt in the coming months. Behind the twelve-year molars are immature wisdom teeth. If you are noticing something else on this X-ray and wondering what that is, it's a set of earrings! We prefer that they are removed for this type of X-ray, but if they were just recently pierced, we'll leave them in place.

Many kids in seventh grade have braces on their teeth. Is this the right time to get started?

When to start braces is a complex question. Traditionally, most orthodontists will start comprehensive orthodontics when all the adult teeth are in—at around age twelve. However, there are a myriad of reasons why early treatment (Phase 1) may be appropriate, or even delayed to a later age. Check out Chapter 9 for more details about braces and orthodontics.

Is there a higher risk of getting cavities during adolescence?

Tooth decay is the most prevalent chronic disease in adolescents and the rate of new cavity formation is highest in this age group. Teens are at a stage in their lives where they are developing and exercising more independence. They have the freedom to make some of their own choices, but sometimes those choices aren't the best for their overall well-being and dental health. Many adolescents will start indulging on coffee, energy, and sports drinks, all with significant sugar sweetening. Additionally, without vigilant parental supervision, adolescents may become complacent when it comes to their oral hygiene routines. The act of brushing and flossing may be of lower priority for a teenager who has numerous other life stressors at the moment, so it's important to re-affirm to them the importance of dental health and how it can be perceived by their peers. Encourage your kids to focus on thoroughness and quality over speed when brushing and flossing. A random "check-in" here and there can be helpful to keep them honest.

Now that my teenager has all their permanent teeth, is fluoride still necessary?

Up until age sixteen, the systemic benefit of fluoride is quite important in establishing a strong enamel structure. Once the enamel of all the teeth is completely mature, the use of additional systemic fluorides, such as through prescription tablets, is no longer necessary or recommended. Instead, it is the topical action of fluoride that will predominantly help to combat tooth decay moving forward. In adulthood, this is best achieved by brushing twice daily with fluoridated toothpaste.

What is puberty gingivitis?

As children begin to go through puberty, their hormone levels fluctuate significantly. Some of these hormones, including estrogen and progesterone, can modify the gingival inflammatory response to dental plaque, making it more intense.[52] This exaggerated response means that the same levels of plaque a younger child may have tolerated without consequence will now cause gingival inflammation in your preteen or teenager. Therefore, adolescents should take their time to perform meticulous oral hygiene, particularly flossing, to prevent gingivitis and its progression to periodontitis. Further details about gingivitis and periodontitis can be found in Chapter 11.

My child's dentist said that we might need a root canal? I thought that was only for old people! What exactly is a root canal and how is it different from a filling?

Recall from our previous discussions that teeth have multiple layers. When the inner layer, the pulp, becomes compromised by bacteria or inflammation, the tooth will require root canal treatment. A *root canal* involves removing the entirety of the pulp. This pulp tissue extends from the crown of the tooth, the visible part above the gum line, down into the root system through thin channels called *canals*. Once these canals have been cleaned out by your dentist, a synthetic replacement material is placed into the now empty spaces of the root. Root canals can sometimes be challenging because some teeth have one root, others have two, and others still have three! After the tooth has finished receiving root canal therapy, the tooth is basically "dead," as it is now devoid of any living tissues.

Why does a root canal-treated tooth need a crown?

Most, but not all, root canal-treated teeth benefit from having a crown placed after the procedure is completed. These teeth have typically experienced a significant loss of structure. Additionally, the procedure has "hollowed out" the tooth of living tissue. A *crown* is essentially a protective shell made of durable materials that encases the remaining tooth, supporting it, and restoring its form and function.

My child lost a permanent tooth early on. Can they get a dental implant?

Dental implants are small devices that can best be described as fancy prosthetic screws. They are typically made from titanium, although other materials such as ceramic are available as well. The implant is placed in the jawbones and functions as the root of a replacement tooth. Connected atop the implant will be a prosthetic crown that acts as the new tooth you see when you look inside the mouth. While implants are the standard of care for lost teeth, there is a unique challenge to consider in children—they are still growing. This is a problem because implants fuse to the bone, a process called *osseointegration*, and can no longer move dynamically as a real tooth would in a growing jaw. As your child continues to grow, the initial site of the implant may look considerably out of place when your child is fully mature. For this reason, dental implants are generally not recommended for children before late adolescence. Many dentists will instead opt to place temporary removable devices known as "flippers" in children who have lost teeth but are still growing. These flippers are reminiscent of partial dentures.

Consider the following case. In Picture (A), two implants are planned to be placed in the green and pink boxes. Both were areas where no adult tooth was present. The tooth seen in the green box is a baby tooth. In Picture (B), you can see the appearance of a dental implant on an X-ray. In Picture (C), the implants have been restored with prosthetic crowns.

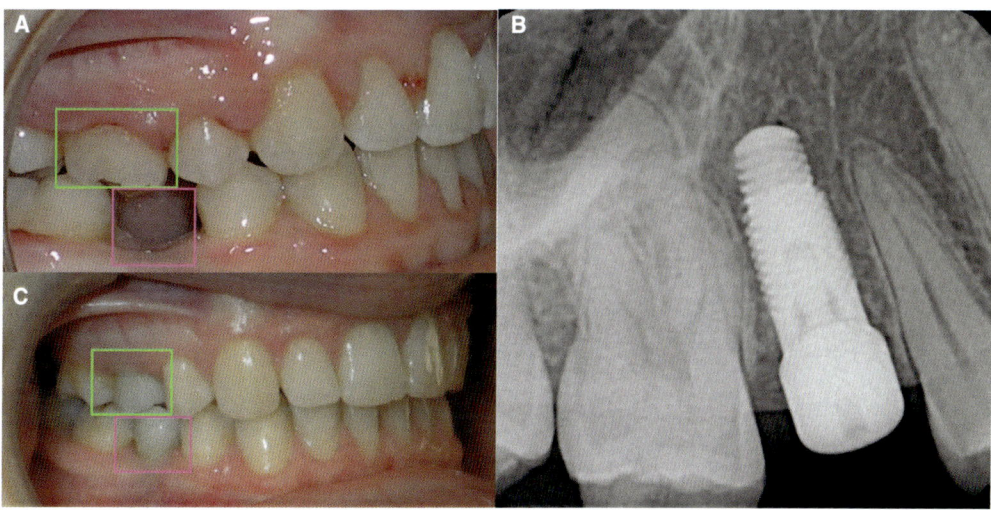

When can my child get their dental implant then?

Your child will be a suitable candidate for getting an implant once their growth is complete. For females, this generally occurs around seventeen-years of age, and for males, this happens a little later, between the ages of eighteen to twenty-one. These ages are only estimates based on reported averages; the exact timing is determined on a case-by-case basis by your dentist or surgeon who may consult growth charts, order skeletal growth films, or assess secondary sex characteristics to make the final determination.

What are wisdom teeth?…And why are they usually removed?

The term "wisdom teeth" refers to the third set of permanent molars that develop all the way in the back of a child's mouth. These *third molars* are the last permanent teeth to develop, and by extension, the last to potentially erupt at around seventeen- to twenty-one years of age. By this point, hopefully your child has gained a little wisdom to go along with their wisdom teeth! Most teenagers however, do not have enough room to fit these teeth in their mouth, but some will be lucky enough to have the space to accommodate them. As a general rule, if the teeth are crowded around twelve- to thirteen-years of age, there likely won't be enough room for the wisdom teeth to erupt when the time comes. The final determination is usually not made until the child is in their late adolescent years. It is important to take panoramic X-rays to check the position of the wisdom teeth to ensure they are not causing a problem with the adjacent teeth, as seen in the accompanying panoramic X-ray. This patient's lower wisdom teeth are undesirably angled in a horizontal direction. Clearly, there will not be enough room for them to erupt, and leaving them unaddressed can lead to potential problems in time. A visit to the oral surgeon is indicated.

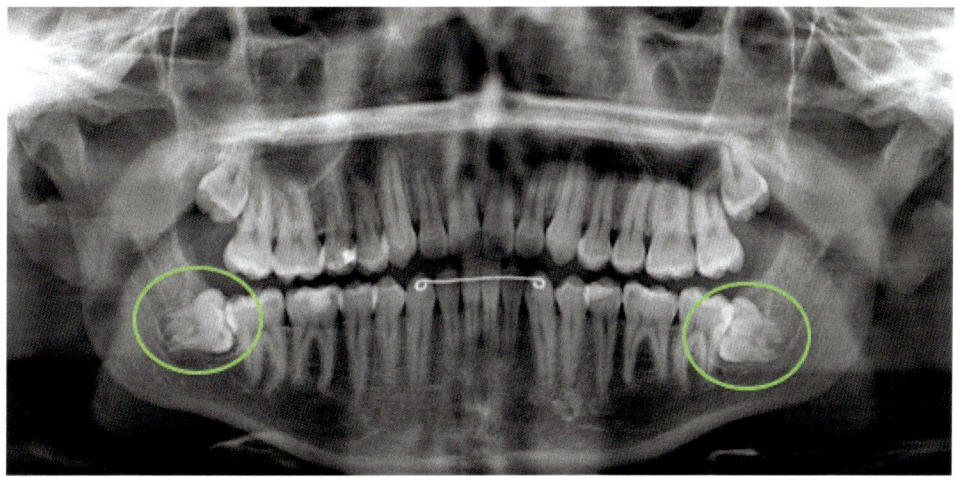

X-ray of a seventeen-year-old. Poorly angulated lower wisdom teeth are circled in green.

In addition to concerns over space, other reasons to remove the third molars may include damage to adjacent second molars, prevention of periodontal issues, cavities in the wisdom teeth themselves, or the presence of associated cysts or growths. Even when these teeth do successfully erupt into the mouth, they can be challenging to care for and keep clean. Most dentists recommend prophylactic extractions before a problem arises if it is obvious there will not be enough room. Removal of these teeth shouldn't be taken lightly though. Any surgery, including tooth extraction can have risks, so there should always be a good reason for removal.

Will the wisdom teeth ruin the alignment of my child's front teeth?

While this is a popular old wives' tale, evidence suggests that a patient's third molars do not heavily contribute to overlap of their front teeth.[53] There are many people born without wisdom teeth whose front teeth still become crowded. Conversely, there are many others with wisdom teeth present that do not experience any crowding at all.

How should I care for my child after wisdom teeth extractions?

Following wisdom teeth extraction, the surgeon will generally opt to place sutures to help close the socket and control bleeding. A soft and bland diet avoiding acidic and salty foods would be ideal for the healing patient. Rice, seeds, and other small foods should be avoided to prevent these objects from entering the tooth sockets. It would also be appropriate to avoid spitting or using a straw during the immediate healing phase, a day or two after the surgery. We wouldn't want to disrupt an established blood clot. Swelling is possible following difficult extractions and will usually peak approximately twenty-four to forty-eight hours after the surgery. Cold compresses applied at about ten- to fifteen-minute intervals can aid in alleviating discomfort and reducing this swelling. While opioid painkillers, like Vicodin, were historically prescribed following wisdom teeth extraction, current data suggests that exposure to these medications in the teenage and early adult years may lead to more chronic long-term inappropriate usage, including substance abuse and dependence.[54] Therefore, a more modern approach to pain management for teenagers with post-extraction pain from wisdom teeth removal is to start with a non-opioid medication such as a higher dose of ibuprofen. This sufficiently manages the discomfort in the majority of the cases. If, however, the pain is excruciating, the surgeon may consider prescribing opioids for short-term use.

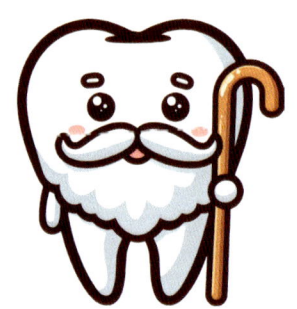

How does one know if their child's jaws are done growing?

Typically, the *mandible* (lower jaw) will continue to grow after the *maxilla* (upper jaw) has finished. Most girl's jaws are done growing between thirteen and sixteen, and most boys' jaws are done growing between thirteen and seventeen. There is of course variation that exists among individuals. That variation is most prominent in people with a "growth excess." For example, children whose bottom teeth stick out further than their uppers due to a large lower jaw will tend to continue growing later into their teenage years, exacerbating the problem. While growth is a very important consideration when planning all orthodontic treatments, it is even more important when there is skeletal disharmony (jaws being either too small or too large). More to come on growth disharmonies in the orthodontic chapter.

How do I know if my child is a candidate for orthodontic treatment?

Orthodontic treatment has a variety of applications and often begins in this age group (twelve- to seventeen-year-olds). On the macroscopic level, orthodontists can manipulate the shape and position of the jaws, and on the micro level, they can subtly move the teeth through rotation and positional changes. For some people, orthodontic treatment is a medical necessity to correct significant bite issues and jaw discrepancies, while for others, orthodontics can provide substantial functional or cosmetic improvements. Almost everyone can benefit from some degree of orthodontic therapy, and this is discussed in detail in the following chapter.

Will my teeth move as I get older?

Absolutely! Teeth will always want to move. The equilibrium of our mouth and face changes as we age, and our teeth move accordingly. Typically, whatever problem your child currently has will slowly get worse without orthodontic treatment and proper maintenance. Therefore, if you have an open-bite, it is likely that the open-bite will increase over time. If you have crowding of your bottom front teeth, it is likely that the crowding will gradually worsen in severity over time. Whatever issue your child is facing, big or small, it will not go away by simply ignoring it.

How can I ensure my child's teeth stay straight?

Since we know that teeth will move as we get older, and we'll all get older with time, this question is relevant to everybody. A *retainer* is the simplest solution to maintain teeth in the desired position. There is a variety of retainer styles out there, and different bites do better with different types of retainers. We will discuss more on retainers in the next chapter.

What is the best option for whitening or bleaching?

Everybody wants that Hollywood smile! Many kids think their teeth are not white enough and want to pursue *bleaching*. It is important to explain that all teeth have a mild tint to them, and most of the time with good oral hygiene their teeth should be within the normal range of brightness. If you do proceed with whitening, the "best" option for your child should take into consideration the cause of the discoloration and your child's expectations. First, one should consider if the color irregularity is on the surface or is deep within the tooth structure. Surface stains, such as those from coffee or tea drinking, will typically respond the best to bleaching treatments. These can be performed with special gels held in place by adhesive strips or trays. Conversely, sometimes the discoloration may be a part of the underlying tooth structure, and in these situations, it may be more prudent to mask the discoloration with a filling rather than try to change its color with bleaching. Review the best course of action with your child's dentist. One should also consider just how bright your child wishes to go, and how quickly they hope to get results. There are different options available for the child who has all the time in the world versus the child who wants their teeth bleached a week before their prom.

Should I use over-the-counter (OTC) whitening products or have it professionally done?

Before buying expensive whitening products we would first recommend consulting with your dentist to make sure your child's goals align with the plan. A consultation can help determine the cause of the discoloration and provide the best options for management. There is nothing inherently wrong with using OTC products appropriately to manage your child's esthetic concerns, and your dentist may be able to recommend certain ones. Whitening toothpastes can lightly polish the tooth surface with chemical or abrasive agents. This is akin to using light grit sandpaper to smooth imperfections from a wooden surface. More noticeable changes can be achieved through bleaching gels, which usually contain some form of peroxide. A dentist can help fabricate custom mouth trays to hold the bleaching material in place, keeping it in close contact with the teeth and preventing accidental irritation of the gums. In some cases, professionally administered fluorescent whitening applications can even achieve noticeable same-day results.

How does smoking, tobacco use, or vaping affect the mouth?

A discussion of all the negative health consequences of smoking could fill a whole other book in its entirety. Suffice it to say, smoking is a strong risk factor for a plethora of medical conditions, both systemic and local, including a host of cardiovascular and respiratory diseases. This has led smoking to be branded as the leading cause of preventable death in the United States.[55] As for the oral and dental consequences of smoking, *oral cancer* can be considered the most concerning. While most oral cancers develop in adults, children and adolescents are not immune, particularly among those who put themselves at risk. The physical and chemical effects of smoking and tobacco products can create permanent genetic changes in the cells of the mouth and set your child up to develop these terrible conditions as the tissue damage accumulates over time. In addition, smoking is one of the biggest risk factors in the development of periodontitis. In fact, smokers are three times as likely to lose all their teeth as non-smokers.[56]

Vaping is the act of using electronic nicotine delivery systems, such as e-cigarettes. According to the CDC, e-cigarettes are the most common tobacco product being used by our youth today.[57] These products may be particularly enticing for adolescents and young adults as they are available in a number of appealing flavors, including fruits, candies, and desserts. While we don't yet know all the negative consequences of e-cigarette use, we can confidently say at this time that children who use e-cigarettes are more likely to use traditional tobacco products and that the solutions contain known eye, throat, and airway irritants like propylene glycol.[58,59] We recommend that vaping products, much like traditional tobacco products, be strongly discouraged.

Nearly nine out of ten smokers start smoking by age eighteen, and 98 percent start by age twenty-six.[60,61] Therefore, now is the ideal time to try and intervene and offer assistance to your teenager to help deal with the social pressures that are at play. If your child has already established the habit, the best results to help them quit are typically seen with a combination of behavioral support and nicotine replacement therapies including patches, gums, and lozenges.[62] It should also be noted just how significantly a parent's smoking habits can influence their children's decision to pick up tobacco. So, if you were ever looking for an excuse to quit...do it for your kid!

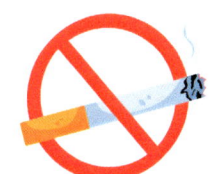

My child wants to get their tongue or lip pierced. Can this affect the teeth?

While these forms of self-expression are popular with adolescents, they are not without risk. There are a number of negative consequences associated with piercings, the most common of which include gum recession and chipping of adjacent teeth or fillings.[63] Tongue piercings typically affect the gums on the backside of teeth, while lip piercings are more likely to affect the gums on the front of the teeth. Less commonly reported issues include the development of speech problems, excess saliva, the development of metal allergies, and nerve damage.[64,65,66] The human mouth is host to many bacteria and thus the possibility of infection should always be considered. If the child is adamant about getting or keeping the piercing, they should ensure the site remains clean and avoid habitually playing with it.

My child has chronic jaw pain. Is this TMJ?

"TMJ" refers to the *temporomandibular joint* which connects the lower jaw to the base of the skull. Each of us has two TMJs, one on each side of the head, and these joints work like hinges that help rotate and adjust the position of the lower jaw to produce its full range of motion. Disorders of the TMJ are known as "TMD" (*temporomandibular disorders*) and can include problems with the joints, bones, or muscles involved in the lower jaw's functioning. While these disorders can develop at any time in life, adolescence is a frequent period for them to crop up, particularly among females.[67]

What can I do about my child's TMD?

Without a definitive diagnosis, it would be best to consider only non-invasive and *conservative therapies* to start with. Physical therapy, like stretching exercises, has yielded positive results in some patients. Behavioral therapy can include avoiding known stressors, addressing tooth grinding, or abstaining from chewing hard foods or gum. Medications, both over-the-counter, like Motrin, or prescriptions, including muscle relaxants and anti-depressants, have also proven effective.[68] A dentist may also fabricate a splint to help balance the way the teeth come together on closure, keeping the jaw in a stable position.[69,70] If your child continues to have TMD issues such as pain in the area of their joint, a professional examination and evaluation by a healthcare provider can help uncover the source of the problem and more aggressive treatments can be considered.

When is the appropriate time to transfer from a pediatric dentist to a regular dentist?

There is no set timetable for when your child should "graduate" to a general dentist. As most children mature, they will feel more comfortable in an age-appropriate adult setting. However, there are some children who will still exhibit behavioral challenges and phobias into adolescence, and these individuals may benefit by sticking with a pediatric dentist a little longer who is familiar with their emotional and behavioral needs. One must also consider the technical work that your child needs when making this decision. In the medical world, we tend to think of pediatrics as applying to children under twenty-one years of age, but in dentistry, your child has essentially lost all their baby teeth and has a full set of adult teeth (excluding wisdom teeth) by age thirteen. With these adult teeth, come different treatment needs, like root canals and permanent crowns that may start to fall beyond the scope of what some pediatric dentists do routinely. Therefore, the decision is best made collectively between the child, parent, and dentist to enable as smooth a transition as possible.

"Whatever." - Every teenager

One-word answers may be a staple of the adolescent vocabulary, but now is not the time to let them give you, or their oral health, the proverbial "brush-off." It may not seem like it in the moment, but despite the eye-rolls and mutterings under their breath, your children will still listen to and respect you. Many adolescents may claim that turning into their parents is their worst nightmare, but hopefully with a kind supportive family that role models good behaviors, in twenty years your kids will look back and realize that it wasn't so bad becoming just like their mom and dad.

CHAPTER 9
ORTHODONTICS

Welcome to the world of orthodontics—where your child's smile transformation begins! If you've ever wondered about the importance and timing of orthodontic treatment, you are not alone. Organized into sections, we'll explore the various aspects of this fascinating topic, making it easier to navigate this subject with confidence. Let's set sail on this voyage of exploration together and discover what role orthodontics plays in your child's life.

1. Introduction to Orthodontics

What is orthodontics?

Orthodontics is the specialty within dentistry that focuses on the diagnosis and treatment of the relationship between the teeth, upper jaw, lower jaw, and lips. Orthodontists aim to improve facial harmony by altering the jaw relationship and the alignment of the teeth.

What is the appropriate age to bring a child for their first orthodontic visit?

The American Association of Orthodontists recommends that a child's first visit to the orthodontist be at approximately age seven. This is a very specific age, as the permanent first molars, those "six-year molars," have either finished erupting into the mouth or are in the process of doing so. These teeth are a *key indicator* that give orthodontists the ability to diagnose various alignment issues more clearly. Most patients seen at this age have no need for treatment yet, but for those that do, this is a crucial time when certain procedures can be performed more efficiently due to bone immaturity and the potential to gain space.

What's the difference between "Phase 1" and "Phase 2" orthodontic treatment?

Phase 1 treatment is considered early orthodontic intervention. It occurs while your child is in their mixed dentition, meaning they have a combination of adult and baby teeth still present. Sometimes this early treatment is referred to as *interceptive* orthodontics. The goal is to literally intercept problems at an early stage before they grow in complexity and become more difficult to manage in the future. This may involve modifying growth of the jaws, maintaining space with an appliance, or selectively removing baby teeth. Phase 2 treatment refers to comprehensive orthodontic treatment— think "traditional braces," when all of the adult teeth are present.

If my child has Phase 1 treatment, does that mean they will also need Phase 2?

Typically, having Phase 1 interceptive treatment will not prevent the need for a future Phase 2. So, what's the point? Well, as stated above, the goal of Phase 1 treatment is to decrease the complexity of Phase 2. This translates to reducing the severity of the problem and potentially the time your child may need to be in braces.

If my child needs braces, how long will it take?

There's no quick and easy answer to this question. While the average child is in braces for approximately two-years, every patient has their own unique challenges that influence the total time required. The length of treatment greatly depends on the original diagnosis and severity of the issue.

Do orthodontists ever remove teeth to make space?

Some patients will simply not have enough room for all their adult teeth. But, how does one know for sure? The answer is found in a simple math equation. On one side of the equation, we calculate the total size of all the teeth. This tells us how much space is required. On the other side of the equation, we measure the size of the dental arch (or perimeter); this tells us how much space is available to work with. In the following two patients, there are different arch perimeters and different degrees of crowding.

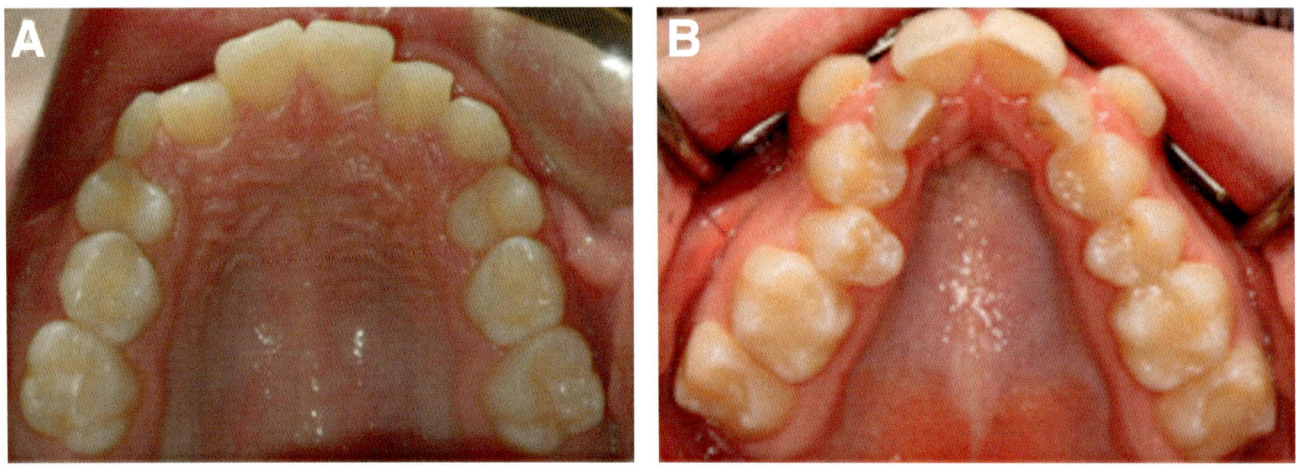

In patient (A), you can see mild crowding of the upper teeth, while in patient (B) there is clearly severe crowding.

The fun of orthodontics is figuring out how to change either of these numbers. Let's start with the arch perimeter. Most of the time we are trying to make this number bigger. With more space, we can fit more teeth into the arch, and crowded teeth have more room to straighten out.

Orthodontists can also manipulate the other side of the equation by lessening the amount of space required. This can be accomplished by filing off small amounts of enamel (known as *interproximal reduction* or "IPR" for short) or by extracting teeth. In example (A), we increased the arch perimeter to provide more space, but in example (B), we reduced the amount of space required by removing teeth.

If extractions are needed to resolve crowding, which teeth are removed?

If the dental arch cannot be made wide enough, extraction of permanent teeth might be considered to resolve a crowding problem. *Premolars* are usually the teeth of choice removed in such situations. Their average size of seven-millimeters makes them appealing, as they are neither too big nor too small to dramatically shift the balance of space. The following photos show an example of a patient who had four premolars removed.

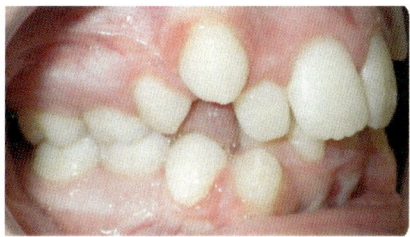 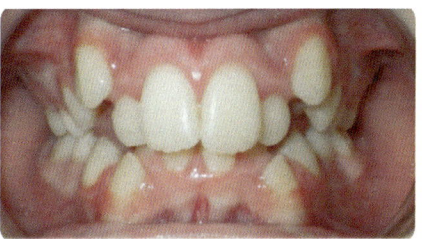 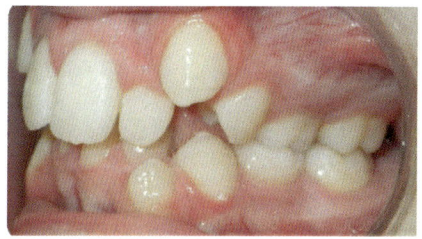

Photos from our initial consultation, where severe crowding was evident. Based on various diagnostic tools, the decision to remove the four first premolars was made to create space to align the teeth in a healthy manner.

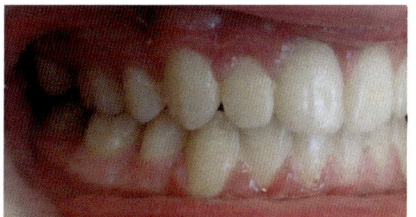 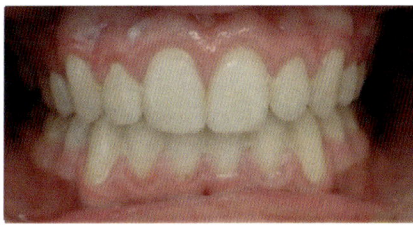 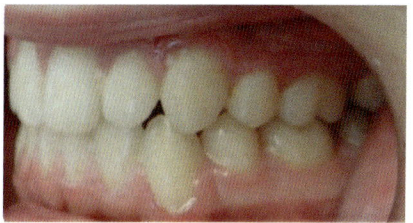

Photos from the day braces were removed. Note the alignment of teeth and highly esthetic outcome.

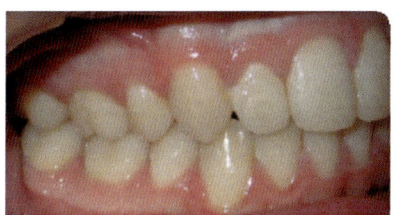 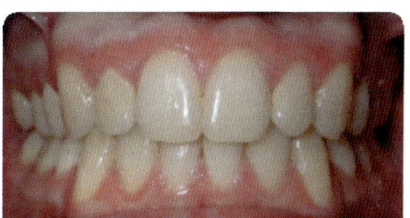 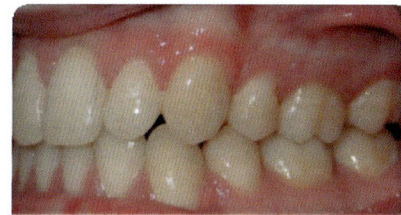

Three years after braces were removed. The smile and bite are well-maintained.

Premolar extractions have gotten a bad reputation over the years. There was a time in the 1980s when they were done far too often, and at times with poor management of biomechanics, leading to unaesthetic facial profiles. When discussing this topic with patients, I will generally tell them, "It is always my goal to treat a case without extractions if I believe I can get an esthetic and stable result. However, if extractions are needed, my objectives include positioning the teeth in such a way that when treatment is complete, no one would be able to tell the difference."

2. Diagnosis

What's the difference between "overbite" and "overjet"?

The term *overbite* is probably the most commonly misused word by parents when it comes to describing their children's teeth. Parents often think that an overbite refers to how far a child's front teeth stick out, but this is not the case! Overbite actually refers to the *vertical* overlap of the front teeth. In other words, it tells us how much the top teeth cover the bottom teeth when closing. Some children have 100 percent overbite, meaning that you cannot even see their bottom teeth when they bite down. The normal relationship is approximately 10 to 20 percent (or one- to two-millimeters) of overlap. The opposite of an overbite would be an *open-bite*, where there is actually a gap between the top and bottom incisors on closure.

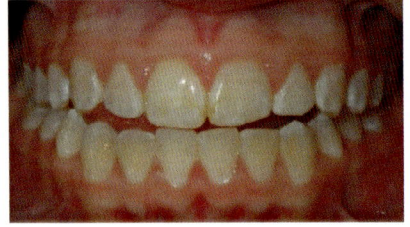
Open-bite

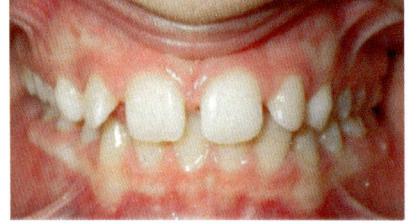
Moderate Overbite

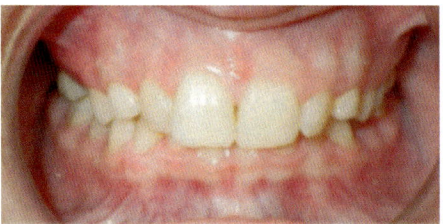
Severe Overbite

Now let's compare overbite to the term *overjet*. Whereas overbite is a vertical measurement between the upper and lower front teeth, overjet is a *horizontal* measurement. Overjet is the true measure that tells us how far the upper front teeth stick out. It's normal to have some degree of overjet; about one– to two-millimeters is considered ideal. The timing and treatment for excessive overjet varies greatly by the severity of the issue. The greater the overjet, the more involved treatment tends to be.

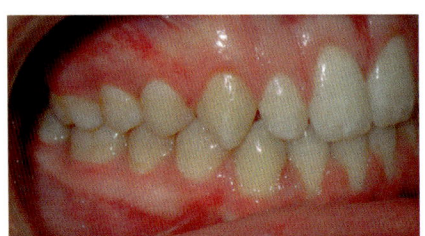
Mild (normal) overjet

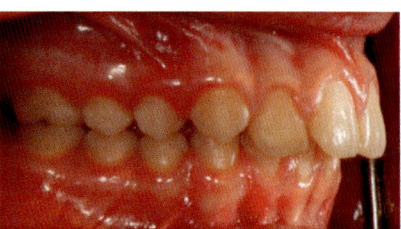
Moderate overjet

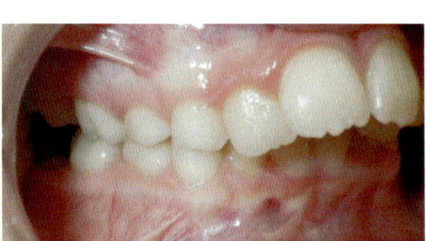
Severe overjet

What about an "underbite?"

An *underbite* occurs when the bottom front teeth stick out further than the top front teeth; the reverse of the normal relationship. Once again, this term refers to a measurement in the horizontal plane. An underbite is a very important finding, and the treatment will depend on its cause. In some people, it might be due to poor angulation or positioning of the front teeth. In others, it may be due to the relative sizes of the upper and lower jaw. The lower jaw may be too big, the upper jaw may be too small, or it may be a combination of the two. The first set of pictures below (A) shows the front teeth coming together in a relationship called "edge-to-edge." This means there is currently no overlap of the teeth and an underbite may develop as the lower jaw continues to grow. The second set of pictures (B) shows a true underbite, in which the bottom incisors are in front of the upper incisors.

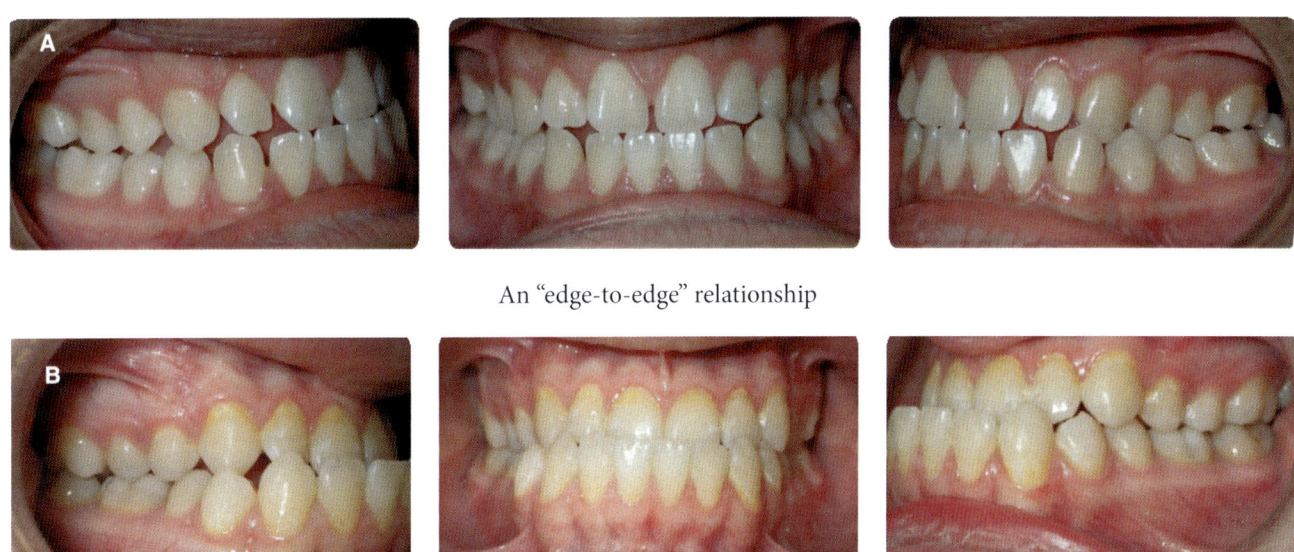

An "edge-to-edge" relationship

An underbite, where the lower front teeth are in front of the upper front teeth.

What is a malocclusion? And what are the different classes?

In an orthodontic context, the word *occlusion* refers to how the teeth come together upon biting down. If the teeth are not coming together properly, it is referred to as a *malocclusion*. Malocclusions can be subdivided into three categories—Class 1, 2, and 3.

Class 1 Malocclusion:

Refers to a bite in which the jaw proportions are within normal limits, yet there are still misalignment issues of some teeth. In this situation, the upper jaw is just slightly forward of the lower jaw.

Class 2 Malocclusion:

Refers to a bite where the lower teeth are set significantly back relative to the upper teeth. This could be due to a variety of reasons, including a large upper jaw, a small lower jaw, improperly angled or positioned teeth, or a combination of any of these factors. This class of malocclusion is often associated with a large overbite and/or overjet. Class 2 malocclusions are most commonly seen in northern European populations.[71]

Class 3 Malocclusion:

Refers to a bite where the lower teeth are further forward relative to the upper teeth. Therefore, a Class 3 is basically the reverse of a Class 2. The causes are the opposite, including a large lower jaw, a deficiency in the upper jaw, improperly angled or positioned teeth, or a combination of any of these factors. This is most commonly seen in Asian populations.[71]

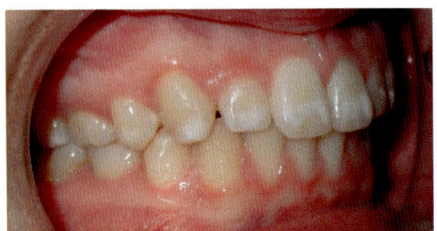
Class 1 Malocclusion

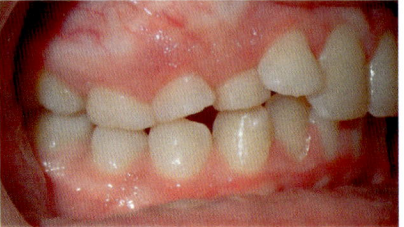
Class 2 Malocclusion

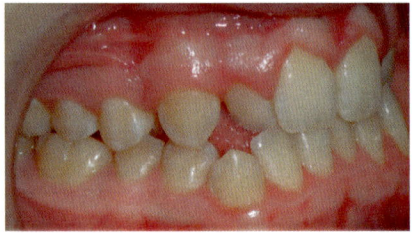
Class 3 Malocclusion

What is "expansion" and does my child need it?

Expansion is the act of widening the dental arch (as seen in the following pictures). It can be done by moving the teeth, known as *dental expansion*, and/or increasing the width of the palate (roof of the mouth), known as *skeletal expansion*.

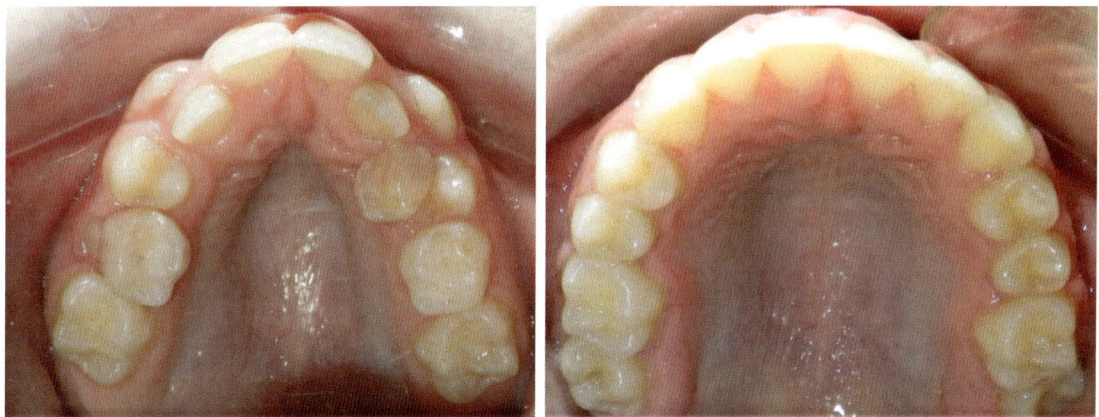

Before and after treatment view of the upper teeth. Dental expansion was used to improve the width of the arch.

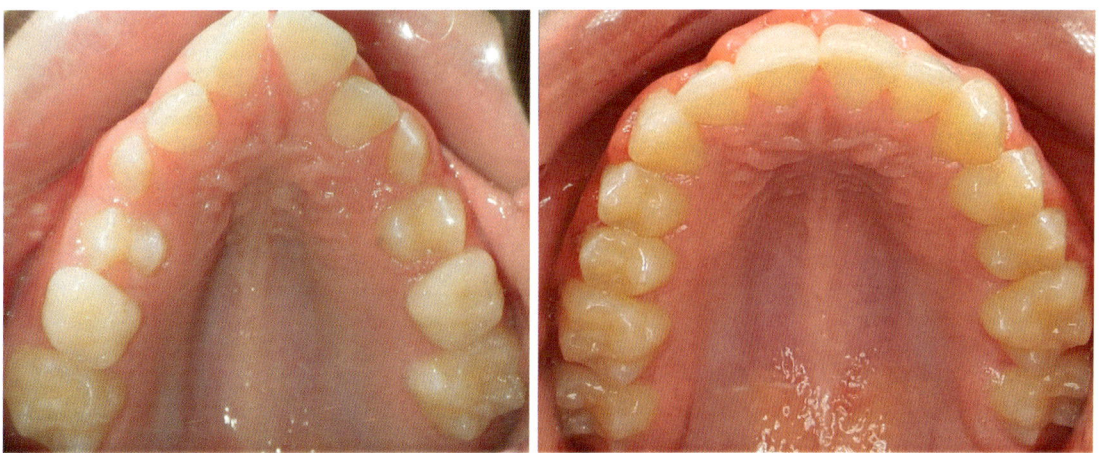

Before and after treatment view of the upper teeth. An expander in combination with braces was used to widen the palate and dental arch.

Whether or not your child needs expansion depends on the relative width of the jaws to one another, and on their spacing needs. For example, the following patient has a crossbite on her left side. A *crossbite* means that the top teeth do not overlap the bottom teeth in the *lateral* (side-to-side) direction. This is a frequent indication that the upper jaw is too narrow, or an asymmetry in the shape of the lower jaw exists. A crossbite on both sides (bilateral) is even more of a reason to expand, as this indicates a more significant discrepancy in width.

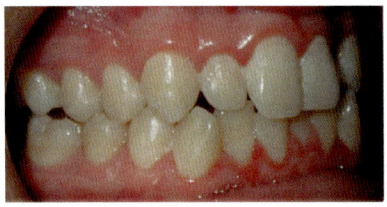 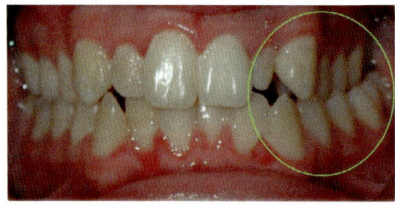 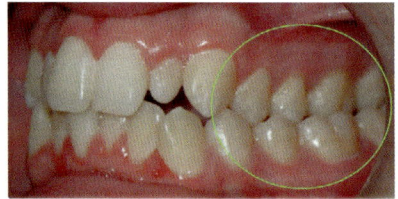

Unilateral crossbite on patient's left noted by a green circle.

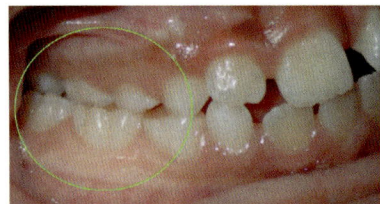 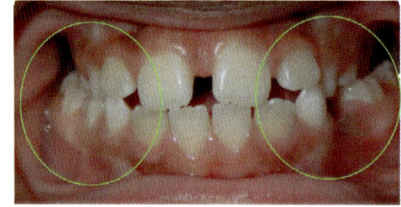 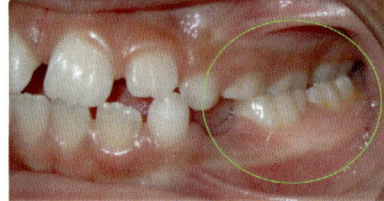

Bilateral crossbite as denoted by green circles on both sides.

Expansion may also be used in the absence of a crossbite, and this may be done to help create space when crowding exists or to broaden one's smile. Of course, there are many factors that orthodontists consider when deciding on expansion and each patient has their nuances.

What is an "expander" and how does it work?

An *expander* is any orthodontic appliance that creates lateral movement of the teeth. Not all expanders are created equal and there are many options to choose from. Certain styles work better for particular bites, and different practitioners have their preferences based on personal experiences and what has worked best for them in the past. Here are just a few examples:

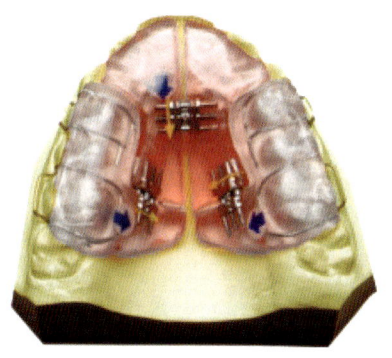 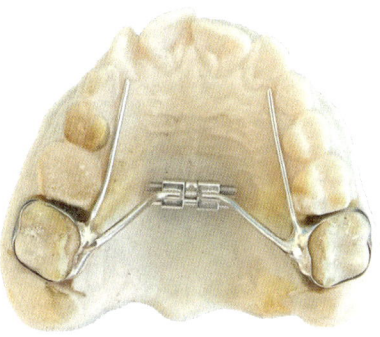 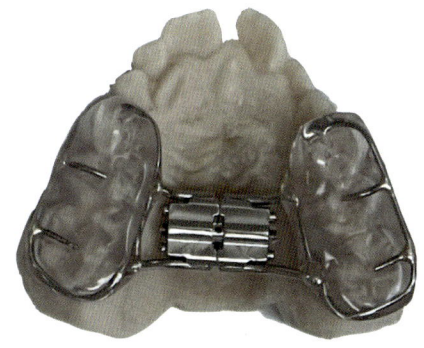

Sagittal three-way removable expander Hyrax rapid palatal expander Bonded rapid palatal expander

Note that all the above expanders are shown connected to models of the upper teeth. Broadly speaking, expansion with an appliance refers to therapy applied to the upper jaw, the maxilla, though there are some exceptions. Most expanders have a *turn-key* mechanism in the center as seen in the examples above. The parent creates a turn by putting a key in the hole and pushing in the direction of the arrow. This turn exerts a lateral force that helps the palate spread apart. As expansion is occurring, it is normal to see spaces begin to open-up between the upper front teeth. This is a sign that things are working, as the teeth are moving further apart in response to the force of the appliance. The amount of visible space created is often based on how quickly the expansion is happening. For example, in *slow expansion*, the orthodontist may have you only turn the expander once a week. However, in a *rapid expansion*, turns may be placed twice a day and wider spaces will open more quickly. The frequency of turns is very important and differs for each case based on the amount of space needed, the type of expander used, and the age of the patient.

Wait...I turn the key?! How am I responsible for helping with my child's orthodontic therapy?

Orthodontics is a team sport. Although the majority of the technical work takes place in the orthodontist's office, the job doesn't end there. As a parent, you'll be responsible for ensuring proper hygiene throughout the course of therapy, helping your child remain compliant in wearing their appliances, and yes, even assisting in the process of moving teeth by making turns in expanders or changing out rubber elastics.

What is the appropriate age for expansion?

Expansion can be done at any age prior to the fusion of the *palatal suture*. Ok...what does that mean? The palate is made of two sections—a right and left half. Note the line going down the middle of the palate in the pictures on the previous pages. This line is where the two halves meet—it is called the palatal suture. As a child matures, the two sides, which were once separate, will fuse together. In girls, this event seems to happen between the eleventh and fourteenth year, and for boys, it occurs between the ages of thirteen and sixteen. As with all age ranges, these estimates are highly variable. Before the halves fuse together, expansion can be performed to spread apart the palate with less force—this is the ideal time to intervene. After the fusion of the suture, expansion is still possible, but it will take more involved methods to widen the arch.

3. Braces

What are braces?

Braces are the small metal or ceramic *brackets* that are glued to teeth. Their function is to enable other orthodontic components, such as wires, elastic bands, or chains, to connect to the teeth and transfer their forces. Let's review the basic types of braces (brackets).

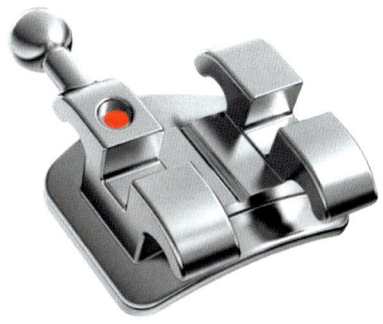

A metal twin bracket –
this one happens to have a hook on it

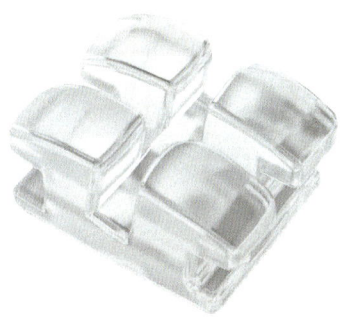

A ceramic twin bracket

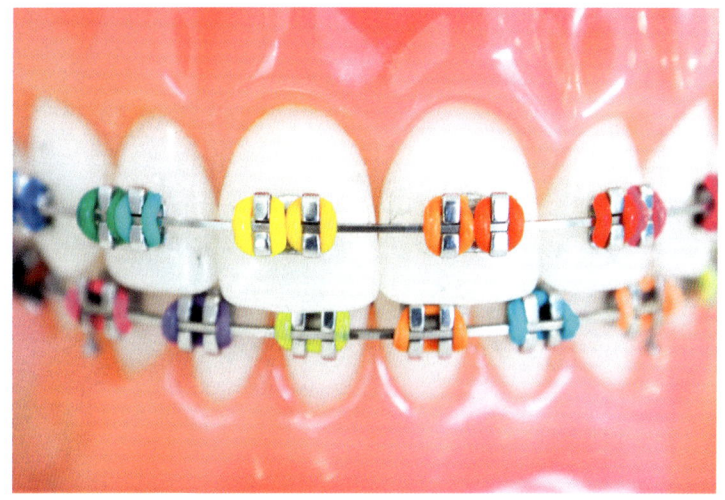

The most common type is called the "twin" bracket. When you see a child with color patterns on their braces, they are generally using the twin style. This type of bracket comes in numerous varieties that differ in size, angle, and the material composition. Metal brackets may be more common, but ceramic alternatives in the twin style are also available and can provide a more esthetic option for patients and children concerned with showing a "mouth full of metal."

A different type of commonly used bracket is the "self-ligating" variety. These braces are designed with a small metal door that locks an orthodontic wire in place without the need for additional accessories like rubber bands. Just as for the "twin" style, so too can the self-ligating brackets be made in ceramics. Though doctors have different preferences as to the type of braces they prefer, all brackets share the same general principles of how they work.

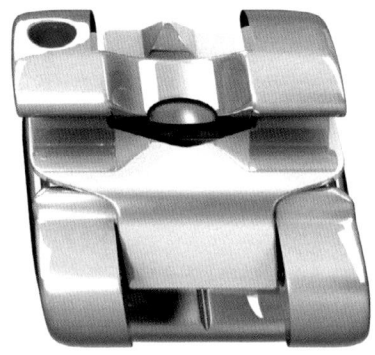 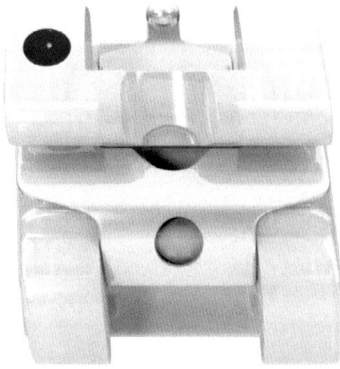

A metal self-ligating bracket, and a ceramic self-ligating bracket.

How do braces work?

The science of tooth movement is a heavily studied topic and there are many textbooks written on the biomechanical "nitty-gritty." Here is the short version—when *forces* are applied to a tooth for an extended period of time, it moves. The direction and manner in which it moves is based on the magnitude and direction of the force, and how it is applied. In most cases, the force comes from the *orthodontic wire*, though other accessories, like elastics, can play such a role as well.

What can braces do?

The combination of braces and wires enable the orthodontist to move teeth to the desired position within the jaws. A tooth can be rotated, pulled up or down, moved right or left, and sent forward or backward. Teeth can move along any of these three planes of space, and this is often why it takes so much time for them to look perfect to our eyes.

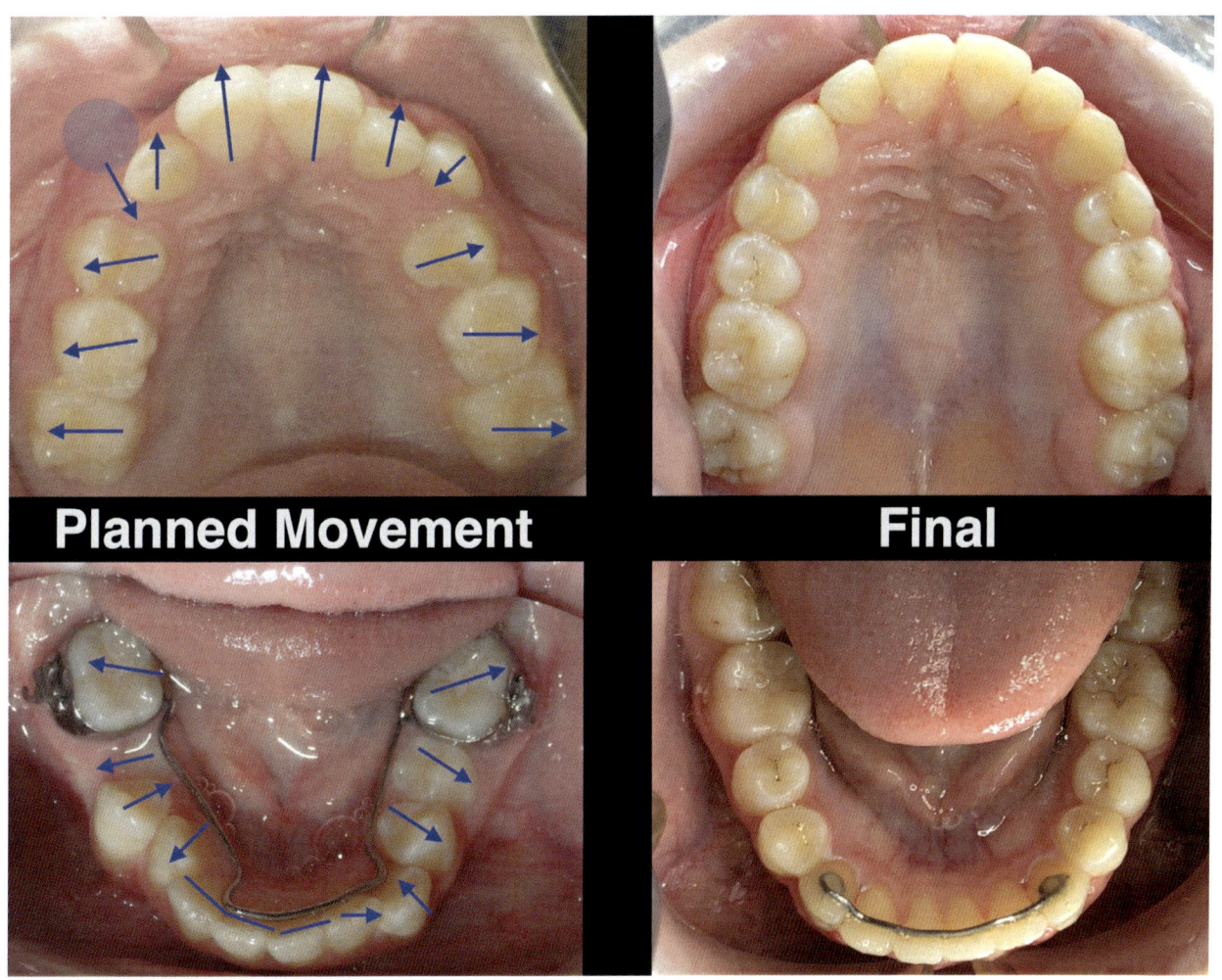

The blue arrows indicate the direction in which the teeth will be moving.
The circle on the top left indicates the canine that has yet to erupt.
The game plan for tooth eruption can be reminiscent of the routes in a football playbook.

How are braces placed on the teeth? Will it hurt to get them on?

Getting braces on does not hurt. Most orthodontists will begin the process by placing cheek retractors in the patient's mouth to help keep the area dry. An adhesive system is used to affix the brackets to the teeth. The precise location and angulation of the brackets is one of the key factors that leads to treatment success. Once the brackets are in the right spot, a specialized light is used to set the adhesive through a process known as *curing*. After the brackets are secured to the teeth, an orthodontic wire can then be *ligated* (attached) with bands, ties, or the brackets themselves. It is the interaction between the wire and the braces that the patient feels. Children most often describe this sensation as "tightness," and it will usually dissipate after two- to three-days. Typically, the first wire is often the one that patients feel is the most uncomfortable. It is advisable to manage their discomfort with the same over-the-counter pain relievers they would use for a headache.

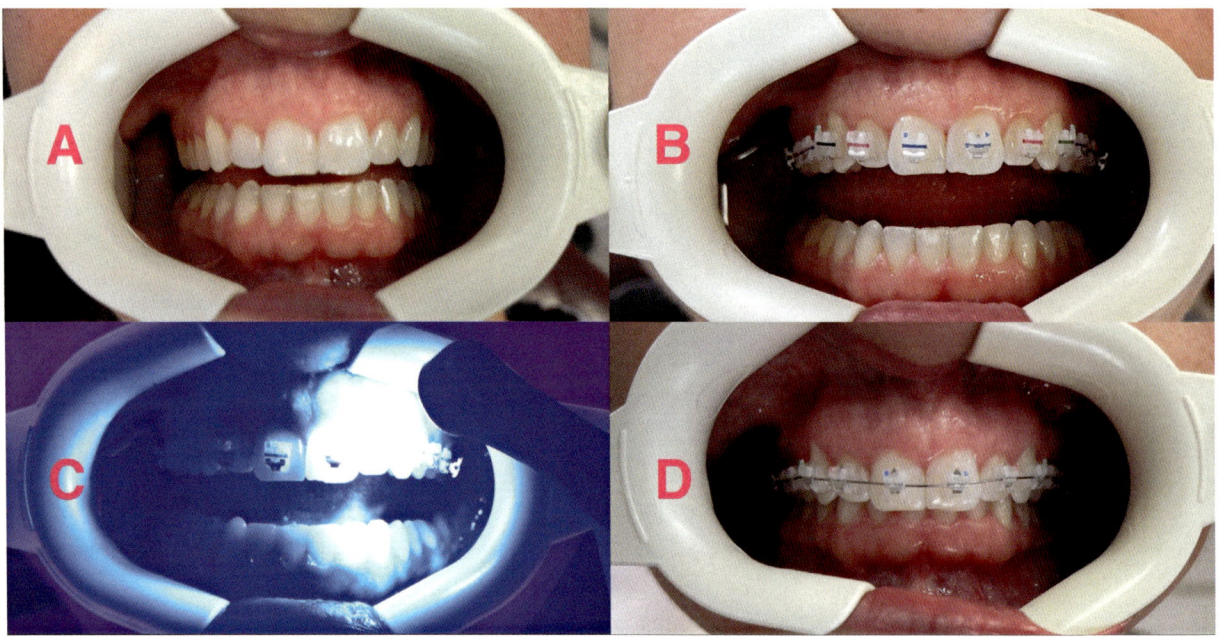

The process of getting braces on. (A) Check retractors are placed to help keep the teeth dry. The teeth are prepared for the brackets. (B) Brackets are placed in strategic positions. (C) A blue curing light is used to harden the glue. (D) A wire is placed, and the braces are connected.

Other than discomfort and soreness, what else can I expect after I get braces on?

Your child may develop a few ulcers or sore spots in response to all the new hardware in their mouth. These sores can either be on the cheek, the lips, or even the tongue. Sometimes these ulcers come and go without obvious provocation, but other times these ulcers are caused by very specific irritants like a poking wire. To manage these sores, we often recommend warm saltwater rinses multiple times a day at the start of braces. The saltwater will not make the ulcer go away, but it will help it heal faster. Certain children who have a history of getting canker sores in their mouth are even more prone to getting ulcers in response to braces.

Patients are often sent home with a care-kit of items on their first day of treatment. Perhaps the most common item in these kits is *orthodontic wax*. Wax can easily be molded to cover any brace or sharp poking wire that is causing irritation in the mouth. Here's a little tip about wax—if you first dry the area you plan to place it, the wax will stick much better!

Is it normal for my child's bite to feel "off" after braces are placed?

Very normal! Our bite is based on how our teeth are positioned, the size of our jaws, and our muscle memory. Teeth will start to move right away after the braces have been placed, and the shifting alignment will cause the muscles and brain to perceive the bite as different.

How is an orthodontic band different from a bracket?

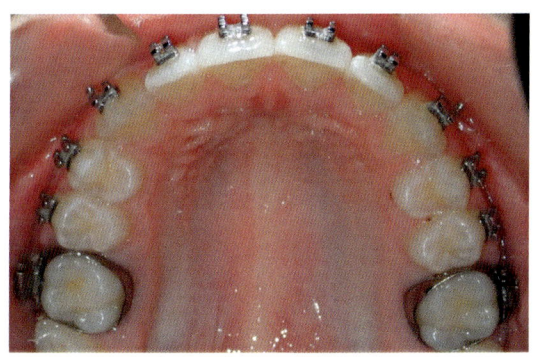

A *band* is a circular orthodontic attachment that wraps around a tooth, similar to how a ring encircles a finger. Both braces and bands are methods of getting a hold of teeth to allow the orthodontist to control their position. Prior to modern braces, every tooth had to have a band attached to guide its movement. This was laborious for the orthodontist and exhausting for the patient…it also wasn't the best of looks. Bands are still used today, though much less commonly; they are mainly reserved for the larger molars in the back of the mouth. Bands can be used as part of expanders, space maintainers, or sometimes to anchor appliances. Band placement also helps to reduce the breakage of braces.

What are "bite bumps" and why are they used?

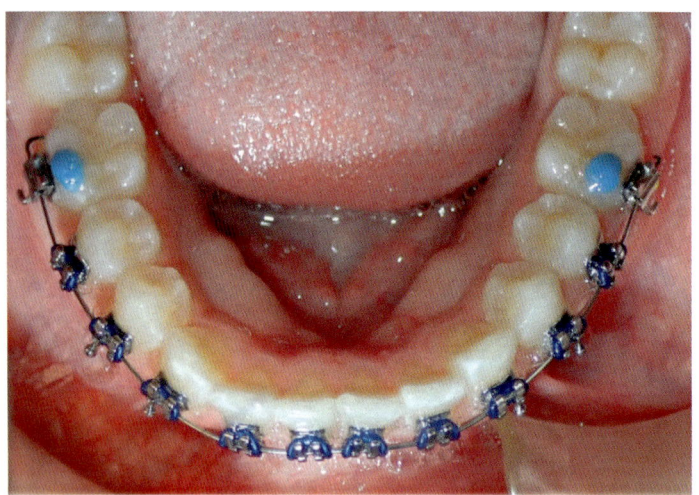

Blue bite bumps placed on lower molars to temporarily open the bite up.

For some children, particularly those with a large overbite, the child's front teeth may hit their bottom brackets when closing. *Bite bumps* are small amounts of resin placed on the chewing surfaces of the back molars to help open-up the bite. By opening the bite, we effectively prevent the patient's front teeth from hitting the bottom brackets and this reduces the likelihood of knocking them off. Most often, these resin mounds are either tooth-colored or bright blue in appearance. When the bumps are initially placed, it is normal for the child to feel as though they are unable to close down all the way…and they are right, that's the idea after all! Over time, the resin naturally wears down, the teeth change angulation, and the bite bumps are no longer needed. Most patients tolerate this well and adjust to the sensation after a few days.

Are bite bumps the same as "bite turbos"?

Bite turbos play a similar role to that of bite bumps—opening the bite. What makes bite turbos different is that they are usually placed behind the top two front teeth rather than on the back molars. Based on the anatomy of the patient, certain practitioners may choose one style over the other.

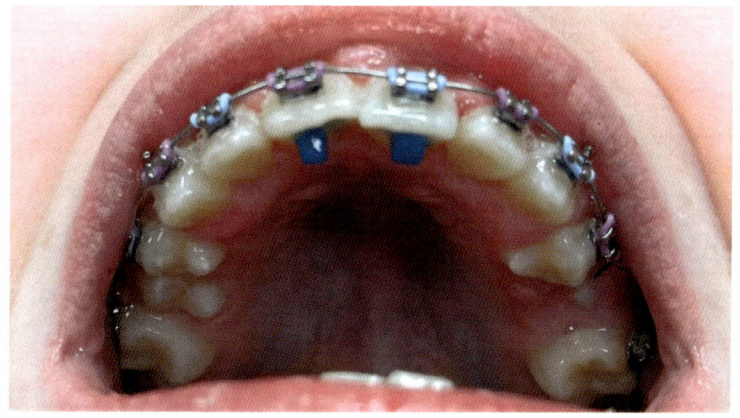
Bite turbos placed behind the upper front teeth to open the bite up.

What if I have a nickel allergy, can I still get braces?

Most metal components used in orthodontics have *nickel* in them to some extent. Stainless steel does and obviously, nickel-titanium does as the name implies. But, do not worry, because there are nickel-free alternatives for braces, wires, and aligners. If you suspect that you have a nickel allergy or sensitivity, it would be wise to alert the orthodontist from the onset.

The American Academy of Dermatology suggests that up to 18 percent of the U.S. population is allergic to nickel.[72] In clinical practice, the number of people seen with allergies seems closer to 2–5 percent. Most commonly, if you have a nickel allergy and make contact with the metal, your skin has a response called *contact dermatitis*, which manifests as a rash with inflammation and itchiness. In the mouth, we call the same reaction *contact stomatitis* and it may present with any combination of redness, swelling, ulcers, white patches, and/or a burning sensation. The surprise nickel allergies usually come from the boys, as most girls will already know if they have the allergic response, having learned from wearing earrings or other jewelry. If your child does have an allergic response to nickel after braces are placed, please give them Benadryl and contact your orthodontist as soon as possible. They will likely remove the brackets and replace them with nickel-free alternatives or reassess for plastic aligners.

What are "elastics" and how do they work?

Elastics are small rubber bands that attach to certain areas of braces or aligners. They play a pivotal role in helping achieve a harmonious bite. Elastics come in different sizes and strengths and can be used in different orientations to exert a force. Imagine stretching out a rubber band…it becomes taught in your hands and the elasticity of the material wants to return to its relaxed state—this is stored energy that can be used to apply a force to move teeth. Let us cover some examples of the most common ways we ask patients to wear their elastics and how this affects the direction of the force.

- Class 2 elastics—Placed from upper canine to lower molar. Helps when there is too much horizontal gap between the upper and lower front teeth. Used to correct excess overjet.

- Class 3 elastics—Placed from lower canine to upper molar. Helps to bring the lower front teeth back or tilt the top front teeth forward. Used to combat underbites.

- Small Triangle elastics—Placed from upper canine to lower canine and first premolar. Used to help "close down" a bite or prevent bite opening.

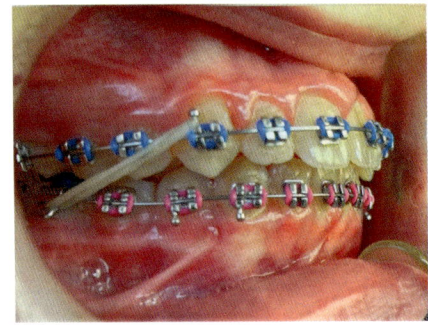

Class 2 elastics from the upper canine to the lower molar

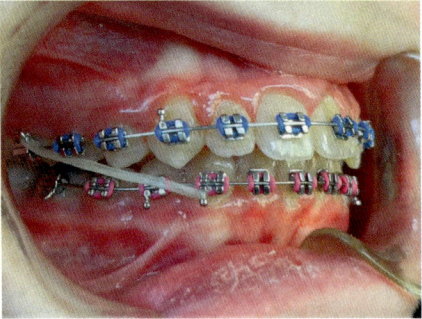

Class 3 elastics from the upper molar to the lower canine

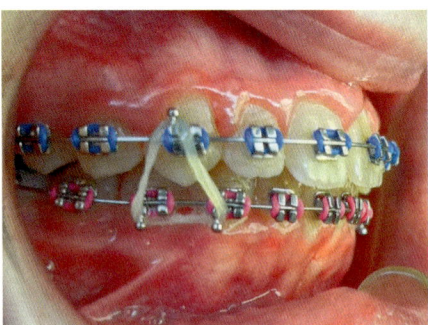

Small Triangle elastics from the upper canine to lower canines and premolars

Let's think about that rubber band again...if you keep it stretched out for too long, eventually it will lose all its springiness and elasticity. Once that happens, the band will have no more force to give and will be useless to move teeth. Elastics must therefore be switched out routinely for a fresh one. This will be the responsibility of the parent or patient to do at home and/or school. It is critical that when your child is shown how to wear their elastics, that you as a parent pay attention as well. The elastics must be connected to the proper teeth, so that movement will occur in the right direction. Being one tooth off might not make much of a huge difference, but connecting them in the reverse manner will apply force in the wrong direction and worsen the problem. For example, Class 2 elastics push teeth in the opposite direction and have opposite goals compared to Class 3 elastics. Therefore, take a picture, or ask your child to take a selfie while at the orthodontist's office, so that you may refer back to it if there is any doubt on how the elastics should be attached.

Will elastics work as well if I only wear them at night?

Wearing elastics only at night will not have the same positive effect as wearing them all the time. This is because teeth *recoil* after moving. At night, the teeth will move in the direction that the elastics are pulling them. The problem is that if you do not keep it up during the day, the teeth will bounce right back, leaving the net change to be minimal. Long story short, the more time spent with the elastics on, the more efficient and predictable the result.

My orthodontist is recommending an appliance to bring the lower teeth more forward. Is that a big deal?

What your orthodontist is describing is a Class 2 corrector. This means there is a discrepancy in the size of the lower jaw compared to the upper jaw, and that this Class 2 discrepancy will not be correctable by elastics alone. Many people fall into this category and it is not uncommon to have to use an auxiliary appliance, instead of, or in addition to elastics, to assist in the improvement of the bite. There are many types of appliances used for this process. They tend to work in a similar fashion, by trying to push the top teeth back, while repositioning the lower jaw and teeth more forward.

What are some things that can go wrong with braces?

One of the most common issues that children encounter is the loosening or breaking-off of a bracket. The term that orthodontists use for this problem is *debonding* and it can occur after eating hard foods, or be the result of a bonding issue with the adhesive used to attach the bracket to the tooth. A debonded bracket is not a major cause for concern, as most will remain attached to the wire and simply dangle in place. If it is the last bracket on the wire, it may slide off and cause the wire to start poking the patient's cheek.

"Pokey" wires are another common occurrence during treatment. Though most orthodontists try everything they can to minimize this, it sometimes still happens. As the teeth start to move and alignment improves, excess slack forms in the wire and this tends to stick out of the back bracket.

What do I do if my child has a broken bracket or a pokey wire?

For a non-irritating dangling bracket that is still secured to the wire, we recommend just leaving it alone and calling the orthodontist's office for an appointment. If it is the last bracket or your child is uncomfortable, there are a few temporary solutions. One option is to dry the area and apply wax over the offending bracket or wire end. Another option is to clip the wire close to the tooth in front of it, where it still remains securely attached. This can be done with either a pair of nail clippers or wire cutters. Just be careful to keep an eye on the part of the wire that you are cutting, so that the child does not inadvertently swallow the clipped end. It's always a good idea to call and update your orthodontist's office to let them know of any issues prior to your child's next appointment. This will allow them to properly set up to make repairs or adjustments as needed.

What are some foods to avoid eating while in braces?

It may sound obvious, but in order for braces to work, we need to keep them intact. Some foods are strong enough to break the bond between the tooth and the bracket. Typically, we tell patients not to eat anything that is hard, brittle, sticky or chewy, but it helps most kids to have specific instructions.

Here is a typical list given to patients of foods to avoid: popcorn, chips, ice, chewy or hard candies, caramel, gum, nuts, pretzels, and crunchy taco shells. If your child loves popcorn, Pirate's Booty is a great kernel-less alternative. Other things that should be minimized, or at least cut into small pieces, include steak, chicken wings, and bagels.

Of course, a healthy diet should still include fruits and vegetables, but if your child is going to enjoy some of the harder varieties like apples, carrots, or corn-on-the-cob, it is preferable to cut them into small manageable pieces and chew on the back molars rather than biting directly into them. Boiling or steaming these vegetables can also soften them up and make them easier to chew. Foods that are easy, tasty, and perfect for braces include soft vegetables, fruits, cheeses, beans, eggs, soft breads, peanut butter, soups, and pasta.

Will braces interfere with my child's activities (speaking, instruments, sports, etc.)?

The answer to this question is "sort of." Kids are resilient, and they tend to adapt to what is thrown at them. While they may be initially guarded in their speech, children will quickly learn to talk with their braces without a noticeable difference in pronunciation. For musical instruments, most kids who play reeds (clarinet, saxophone, etc.) do not struggle with the change. The horns (trombone, trumpet, etc.) however, may take a little longer getting used to, as kids pucker to play them. Their braces will rub against the inside of their lips, causing irritation that may lead to oral ulcers. Remember that saltwater rinses play a significant role in helping prevent and heal these sores.

The biggest difference braces will create for athletes is in regards to mouthguard usage. Many sports, such as football and hockey, now require their athletes to wear them. Children in braces will need to ensure the mouthguard fits around the brackets, wires, or other accessories. These mouthguards tend to be bulkier and are therefore a little less comfortable to wear. We typically recommend the "Shock Doctor for Braces" brand. With any of the options on the market, it is important to make sure they are advertised as "for braces."

4. Non-traditional Braces Options

What about aligners? Is my child a candidate for Invisalign® or a similar aligner system?

A tooth does not know what is pushing it; it could be a metal bracket and wire, or it could be a plastic aligner. *Aligners*, also known as trays, are retainer look-alikes that move teeth by forcing small positional changes upon them. Over the course of therapy, a patient will go through a series of different trays, each shaped progressively closer to the desired final alignment. You can think of each aligner as representing a sequential checkpoint as the teeth move from their starting spot to the finish line. Generally, each aligner is worn for about one- to two-weeks before being switched out for the next in the series. When first trying in a new aligner the patient will feel as though it is quite tight. Once again, this tightness is the result of forces pushing the teeth into the desired position. By the time the patient is ready for their next tray, the aligner will fit more easily since the teeth have reached the next checkpoint and the forces are no longer present. Aligners provide an esthetic and potentially more hygienic approach to orthodontics. Their greatest benefits are that they are nearly invisible and they can be easily taken in and out to brush and floss one's teeth. The biggest drawback however, is that they require very strict compliance to work properly. For example, when a patient starts treatment,

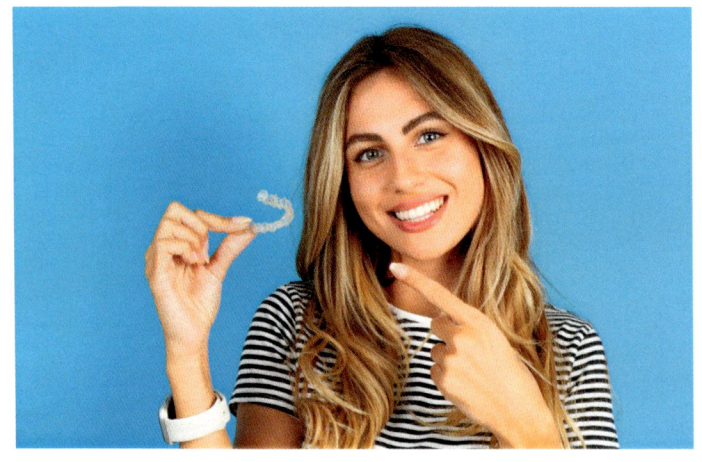

it is recommended that they wear the aligners for twenty-two hours per day. What that really means is the child should wear them all the time, except when they are eating. Ideally, they should brush, or at least rinse, prior to putting them back in. If the patient only wears the aligners at night versus full-time, the results are going to be drastically different. Some children and teenagers can handle this responsibility, but many cannot.

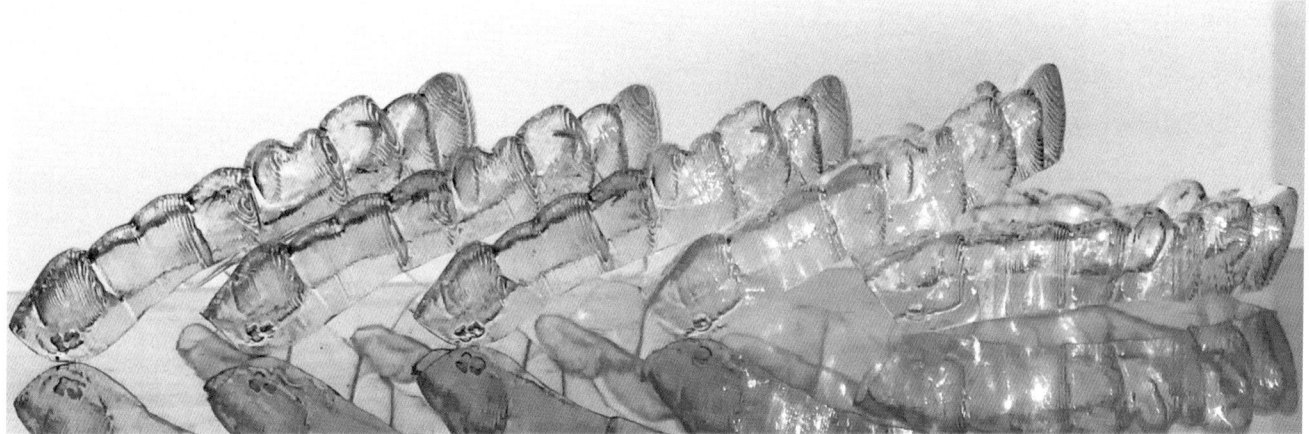

A series of five aligners.

Certain types of bites work well with aligners while others are easier to correct with braces. Combining the orthodontic diagnosis with the parent's knowledge of their child's level of responsibility helps to answer the question of whether aligners are a good fit for your child.

How do you keep aligners clean?

It is important to maintain clean aligners throughout the course of therapy. They can easily pick up food debris, leading to stains, odors, and an increased risk of cavities. Try to build the habit of brushing the aligner every time the teeth are brushed, which is hopefully after every meal. Retainer cleaners (e.g., Retainer Brite) are also good methods to help keep aligners clean. They work similarly to a denture cleaner—place a tablet in a glass of water, drop in the aligner, let it soak, and sit back as the magic happens.

What about braces on the inside of the teeth? What are those about?

Braces on the inside of the mouth are known as *lingual braces*. As with aligners, this treatment has gained popularity as an esthetic alternative to traditional braces. Check out this example of a patient wearing InBrace lingual braces (InBrace is one of the companies that makes them). As you can see, they are glued to the backside of your teeth, and they are not visible at all from the front. Note that there is still a wire that connects all the brackets together. Lingual braces are more common in adults, but once all the permanent teeth are in place, this treatment becomes an option for teenagers as well. Especially for those that do not want visible braces or the compliance of aligners. Discuss with your orthodontist if you want to learn more about this approach.

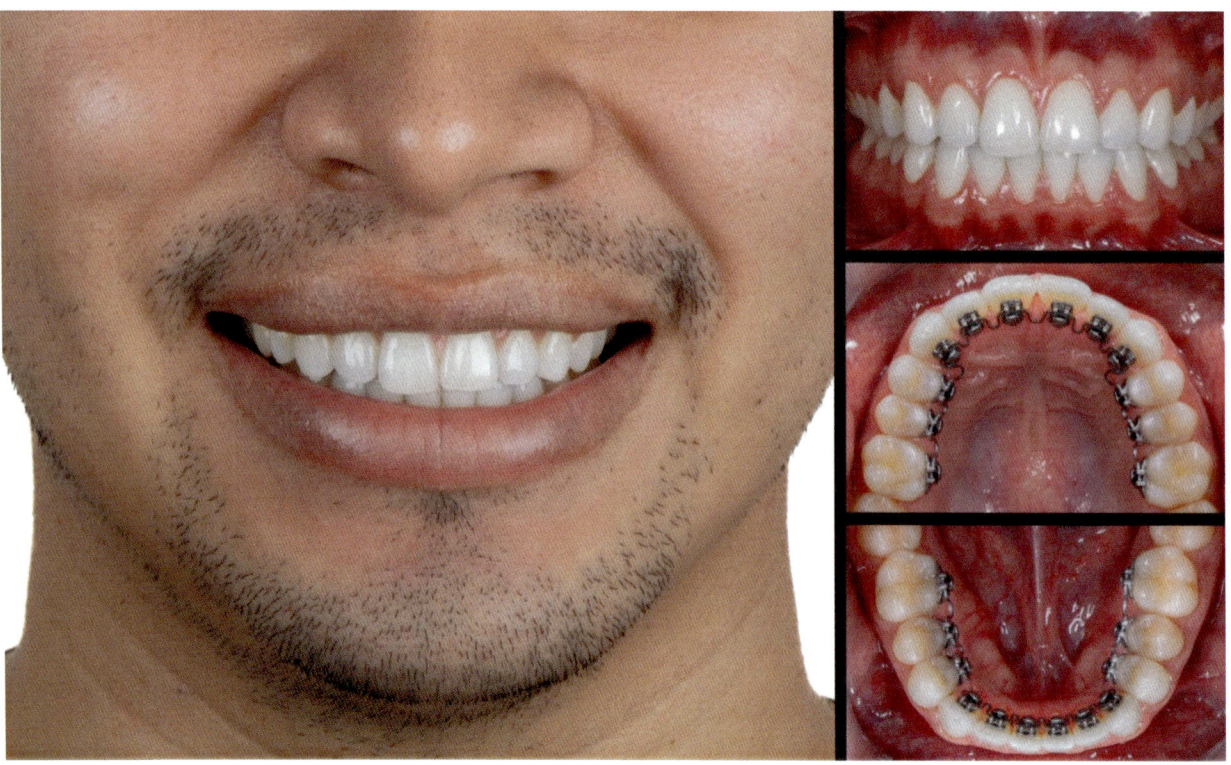

A patient in InBrace lingual braces.

5. Oral Hygiene During Orthodontics

If we're going to the orthodontist, do we still need to see the regular dentist every six-months?

Most definitely! Braces are "plaque traps," food and bacteria can easily get stuck between them and the teeth. Braces automatically put your child at a higher risk for getting cavities and so we need to make sure those teeth stay extra clean. While most people see their dentist twice annually for check-ups and cleanings, we encourage adding an extra visit to increase the frequency to once every four-months for those in braces.

Does my child need to brush their teeth more often with braces on?

Without question they do! Plaque adheres to braces (and other orthodontic appliances) much more easily than natural tooth structure, and therefore your child will correspondingly need to brush much more frequently. Not only that, but braces can make tooth brushing and flossing more difficult. Imagine trying to scrub your teeth clean but there's a metal wire in the way. Oral hygiene is always important...but while in braces, it becomes super important. Those with braces should aim to be brushing at least four times a day, more or less after every meal, at wake-up, and before bedtime. For every patient undergoing orthodontic treatment, we recommend a high-fluoride prescription toothpaste. PreviDent 5000 or the generic equivalent is our preference and should be used once daily at bedtime. This recommendation is intended to help fight decay and minimize the development of unsightly tooth decalcifications known as "white-spots." The same hygiene rules apply to removable orthodontic appliances such as retainers or aligners.

    It is often asked if you have to be gentler while brushing your teeth with braces. If brushing is done properly, there should be no concern in terms of doing any damage to the braces or wires. It is important to pay extra attention to detail, as the whole tooth and bracket should be brushed. This means angling the toothbrush to get to the hard-to-reach areas. Counting each tooth while brushing is a trick that helps many people ensure that no tooth is left behind.

My child got their braces off and now has white spots. What are those and can they be fixed?

The next photo highlights the potential development of chalky white spots around an area where the braces were attached. White spots represent the very first signs of a cavity. In this early stage, demineralization of enamel has occurred but the actual tooth structure hasn't collapsed yet.[73] These spots can range in size, sometimes being quite noticeable with braces on, while at other times, they might only become evident once the braces are removed and the tooth surface can be viewed clearly. Nobody wants to see white spots on their child's teeth, especially after the time and effort spent improving their smile. Nevertheless, if hygiene is poor throughout treatment, white spots are almost a certainty. This is one of the reasons why orthodontists harp and emphasize the significance of maintaining excellent oral hygiene. A child may not be upset about their white spots in the moment, but in time, they will inevitably regret it.

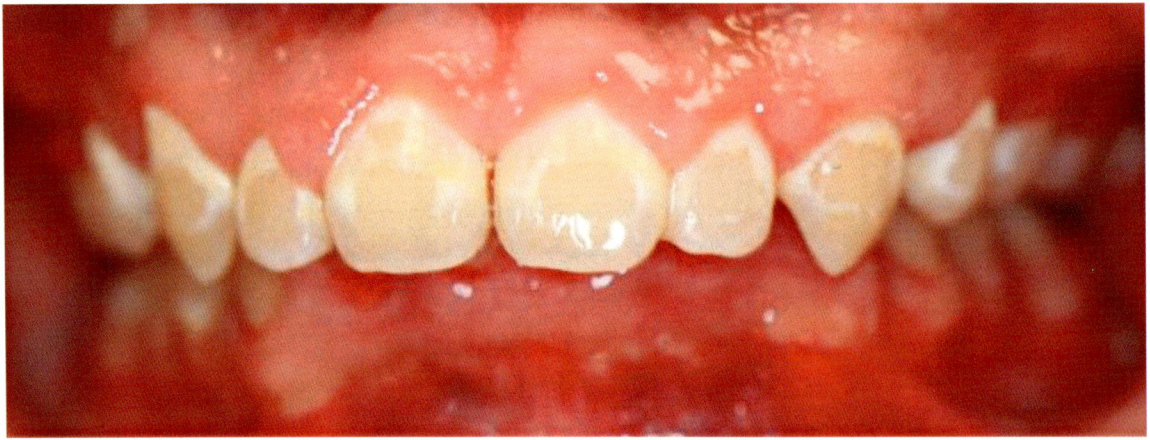

White spots seen on many of the teeth due to poor oral hygiene.

Once white spots exist, they typically do not disappear on their own. The first line of therapy is something called *MI paste*. It is a calcium-containing paste that is brushed or placed on the teeth overnight. The goal of the MI paste is to prevent the white spot from getting worse and to help blend the defect into the adjacent enamel. Be aware that there is a milk-related protein in MI paste, so it should not be used if your child has a milk allergy. If the white spots are still prominent, the next step would be to discuss restorative treatment options with the dentist.

If my child has bad oral hygiene or gets frequent cavities, should they even get braces?

It may be difficult to accept, but if your child struggles with a mouth full of tooth decay or visible dental plaque, it is better not to get braces on until they are mature enough to handle the responsibility. Braces require a rigorous oral hygiene routine and the failure to follow through will only lead to irreparable harm to their permanent teeth. Most teens want braces to improve the cosmetic appearance of their smile, not worsen it. It's one of the worst feelings in dentistry when we remove braces at the end of treatment and find the child has numerous new cavities because they did not take oral hygiene seriously. Worse yet, we don't even make it to the end of treatment because the situation has gotten so bad that we need to take the braces off midway through therapy. However, do not despair! If your child really wants braces, use this as an opportunity to motivate them to improve. Let them demonstrate to you that they can indeed keep their teeth clean and go cavity-free at their next check-up, then they can earn a referral to the orthodontist.

6. Other Important Things

I've heard stories about headgear. Is it still used?

Orthodontic *headgear* has gotten a bad reputation over the years, often conjuring up images of medieval contraptions that look like torture devices. However, headgear is certainly still used when appropriate. There is geographical variation to this and younger practitioners seem to be favoring headgear less than some of the older orthodontists. Headgear is an *external* apparatus, worn partly out of the mouth that connects to the upper molars.

In patients with a predisposition to an underbite, *reverse-pull* headgear is used to help bring the upper jaw and its teeth forward. Elastics are connected from the inside of the mouth to the external apparatus as seen in the photo.

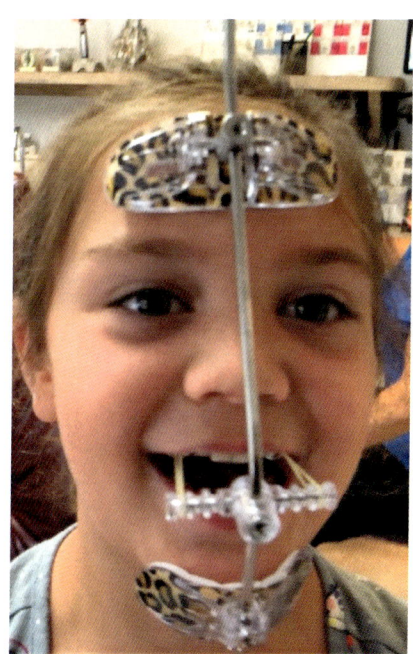

Seven-year-old wearing reverse-pull head gear to help pull the upper teeth forward.

Different styles of headgear can be used for the opposite movement, to pull the upper molars back or to restrict forward upper jaw movement. *High-pull* or *cervical-pull* headgear accomplishes this goal. The most difficult aspect of headgear is typically compliance. The external appliance can often be cumbersome, cosmetically off-putting, and not fun to wear. However, when worn properly and for enough hours, headgear can move teeth impressively.

My child is still sucking their thumb and can't seem to quit. What are the options?

As discussed in previous chapters, habits such as thumb sucking can have long-lasting negative effects on jaws and teeth if not dealt with at an early age. Thumb sucking treatment usually starts conservatively and gets more involved depending on the age of the patient and magnitude of the problem. If you are having trouble stopping it, we are going to presume you have already tried the conservative approaches to therapy such as addressing motivation, providing verbal correction, and using positive reinforcement (like a reward calendar). A non-invasive step up from these techniques may include physical accessories like using a thumb guard or gloves to block the finger from entering the mouth. One additional option to consider is a nail polish called Mavala. It's painted on the nail bed and the bitter taste can be effective in discouraging the child from sucking their thumb. If all these therapies fail, there are various orthodontic appliances that can be used. Traditionally, very intrusive devices were made and placed on the roof of the mouth with prongs or spikes to make contact with the thumb uncomfortable. This technique is still used, but often as a last resort. A similar but less intrusive appliance is called a tongue tamer. Commonly used to prevent a tongue thrust, a tongue tamer can be bonded on the backside of a front tooth where the thumb wants to make contact. The great thing about tongue tamers is that when the child smiles, they are not visible to anyone so the therapy can be performed discretely and decrease self-consciousness. In the photos on the next page, you can see an eleven-year-old with an active thumb-sucking habit. Open-bite and excess overjet are both present, which is common for these patients. Tongue tamers were placed on the backside of the front teeth, which created a reminder to not suck the thumb and to keep the tongue back.

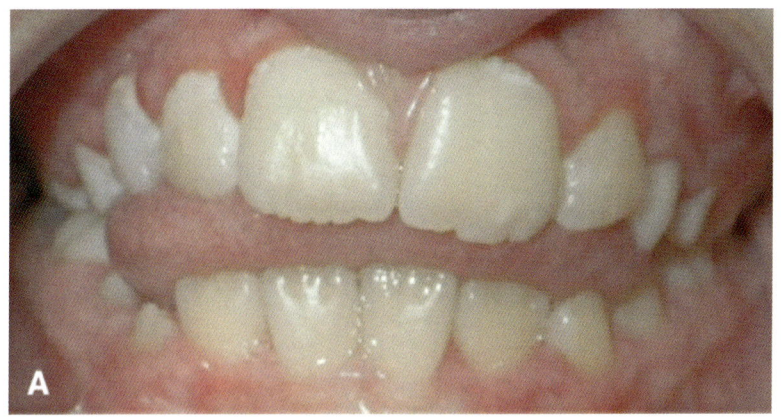

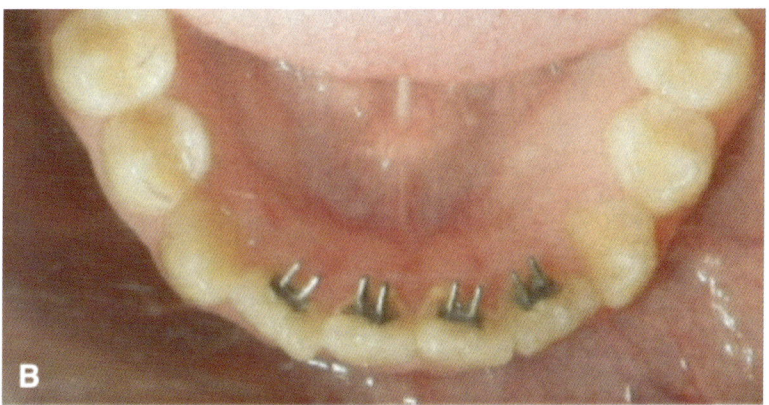

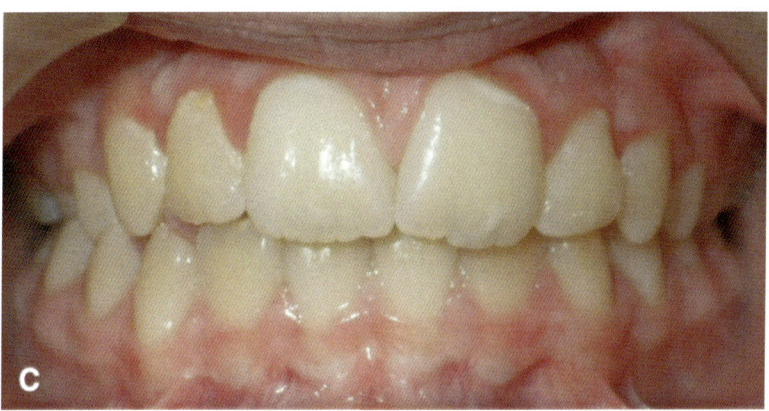

Picture (A) is an 11-year-old field hockey player who presented with an open bite of her front teeth. Tongue tamers were placed on upper and lower front teeth as seen in picture (B). Nine months later, significant improvement of the open bite is seen in picture (C).

What is a tongue thrust?

Our tongue plays a critical role in chewing, swallowing, and talking. The tongue is also one of the strongest muscles in the body. At rest, the tongue should lay toward the roof of the mouth with the tip near the top front teeth. Upon swallowing, the tongue should move to the floor of the mouth.

When pushed too far, even a strength can become a weakness. A *tongue thrust* occurs when the muscle inappropriately moves forward between the front teeth upon swallowing, instead of going toward the floor of the mouth. Often patients with an open-bite tend to have a tongue thrust; but does the open-bite lead to a tongue thrust or does the tongue thrust lead to an open-bite? That's a "chicken or the egg" type of question. Nevertheless, this is why creating overlap of the front teeth is such an important objective of treating open-bites. Once overlap of the front teeth is achieved, many tongue thrusts tend to dissipate.

What is a "smile arc" and "smile line"?

A *smile arc* refers to how one's upper teeth relate to their lower lip. In an ideal smile, the edges of the upper teeth would parallel the curvature of the lower lip. While some people are born with this symmetrical pattern, most are not so lucky.

The *smile line* refers to the amount of upper front teeth you show when you smile. If the upper lip covers most of your teeth when smiling, you are considered to have a low smile line; conversely, if you show all of your teeth and a lot of gingiva upon smiling, this would be a high smile line, also known as a *gummy smile*. Ideal esthetics would have the upper lip resting just above the upper incisors when smiling. It is the goal of the orthodontist to improve these relationships, but sometimes, anatomic limitations prevent perfection. In the accompanying photos, you can see a teenager who, prior to orthodontic treatment, had a low smile line and a flat smile arc. After completion of orthodontics, the teeth were moved in such a way that his smile changed both in terms of how much the teeth were visible on smiling (smile line) and where the edges of the teeth paralleled the lower lip (smile arc).

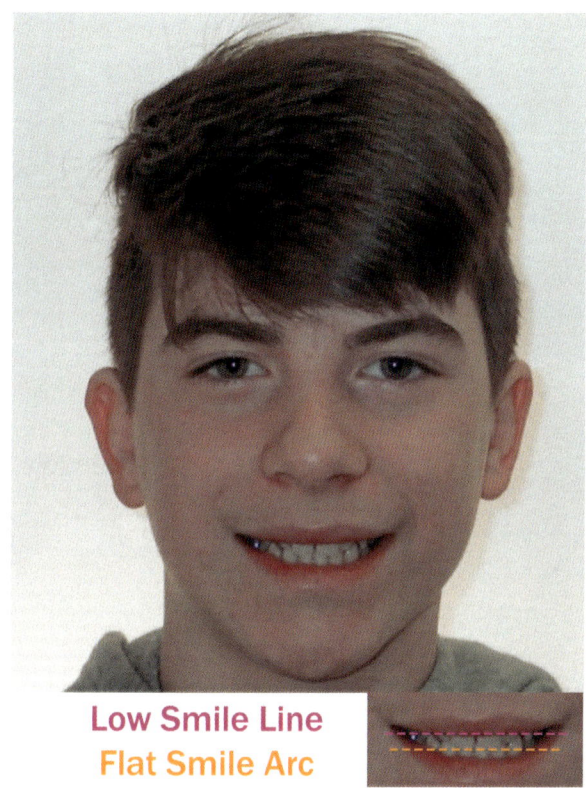 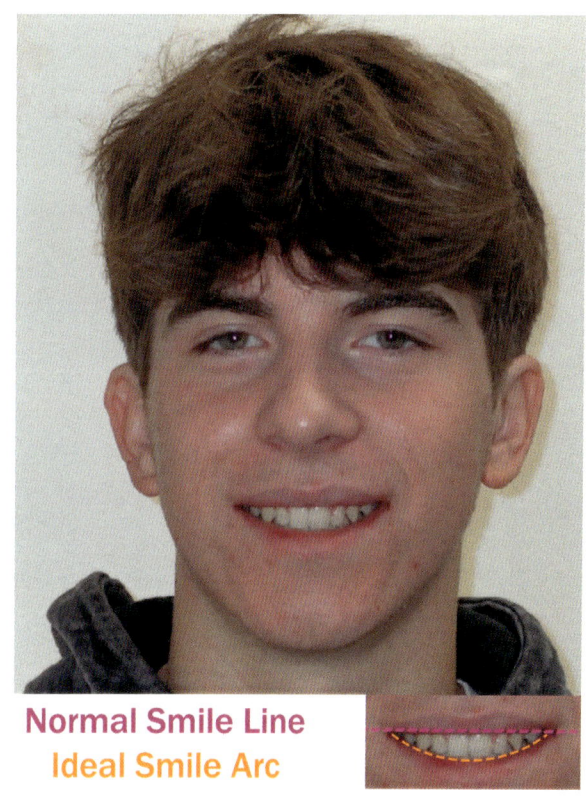

Low Smile Line
Flat Smile Arc

Normal Smile Line
Ideal Smile Arc

Changes to the smile go a long way in improving esthetics.

Is it possible to outgrow orthodontic treatment?

"Outgrowing treatment" means that certain orthodontic problems cannot be permanently corrected while the child is still in their growing phase despite early intervention with braces and appliances. Patients who have a Class 3 disposition, or underbite tendency, are the ones most likely to outgrow their treatment. For this reason, often a full set of braces is not rushed if an underbite is already visible, or if there is a family history of such a problem. In these instances, orthognathic surgery in combination with orthodontics may be the only option to achieve the desired result.

What is orthognathic surgery?

Orthognathic surgery is a procedure in which the jaws are manually repositioned and/or altered in size and shape to harmonize the face and correct a misfitting bite. These procedures are usually completed by an oral and maxillofacial surgeon. There are multiple indications for orthognathic surgery: too large or small of a lower jaw, too large or small of an upper jaw, too long or short of a face, or a large asymmetry or crooked jaw. Though a very involved surgery and recovery, this procedure typically has a profound impact on the patients that undergo it. The following photos are an example of how the surgery can drastically change someone's bite and smile.

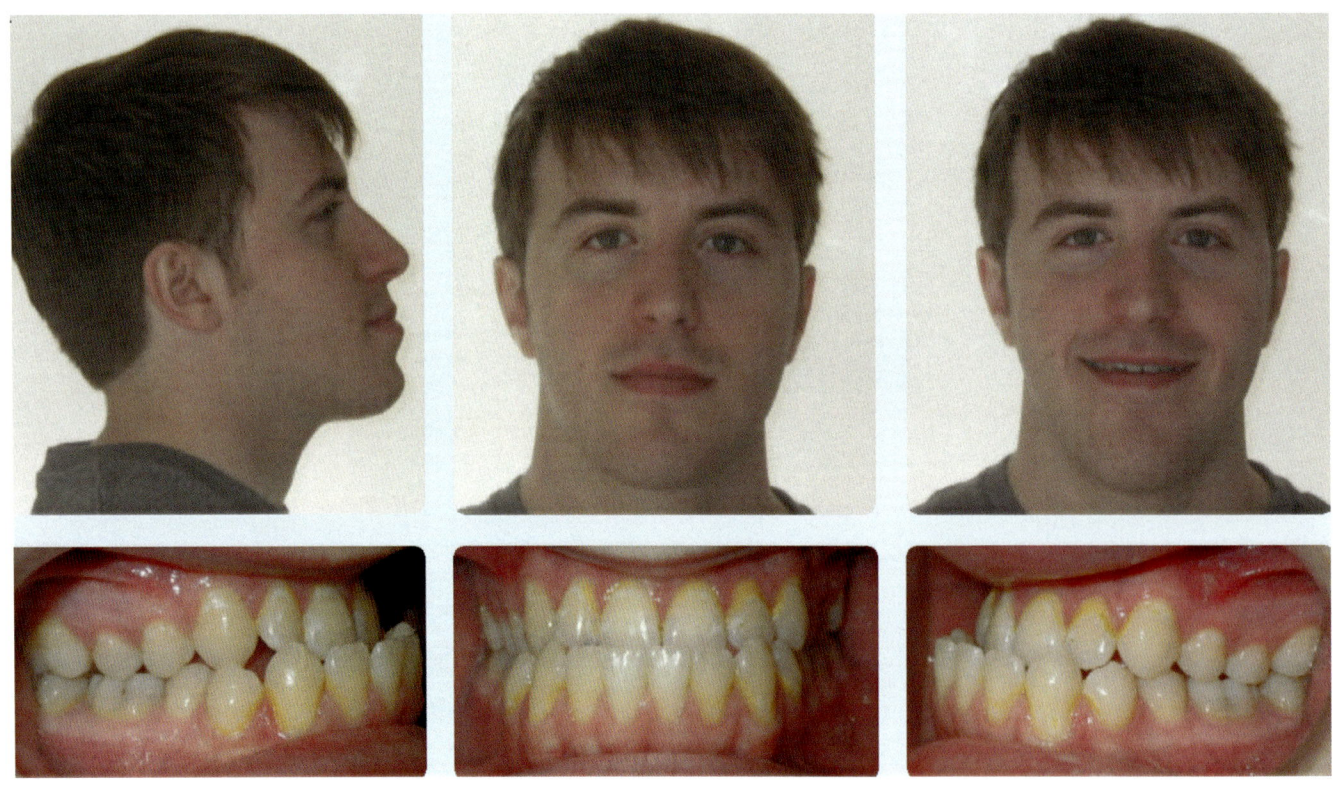

Pictures show a patient with an underbite that cannot be corrected with orthodontics alone.

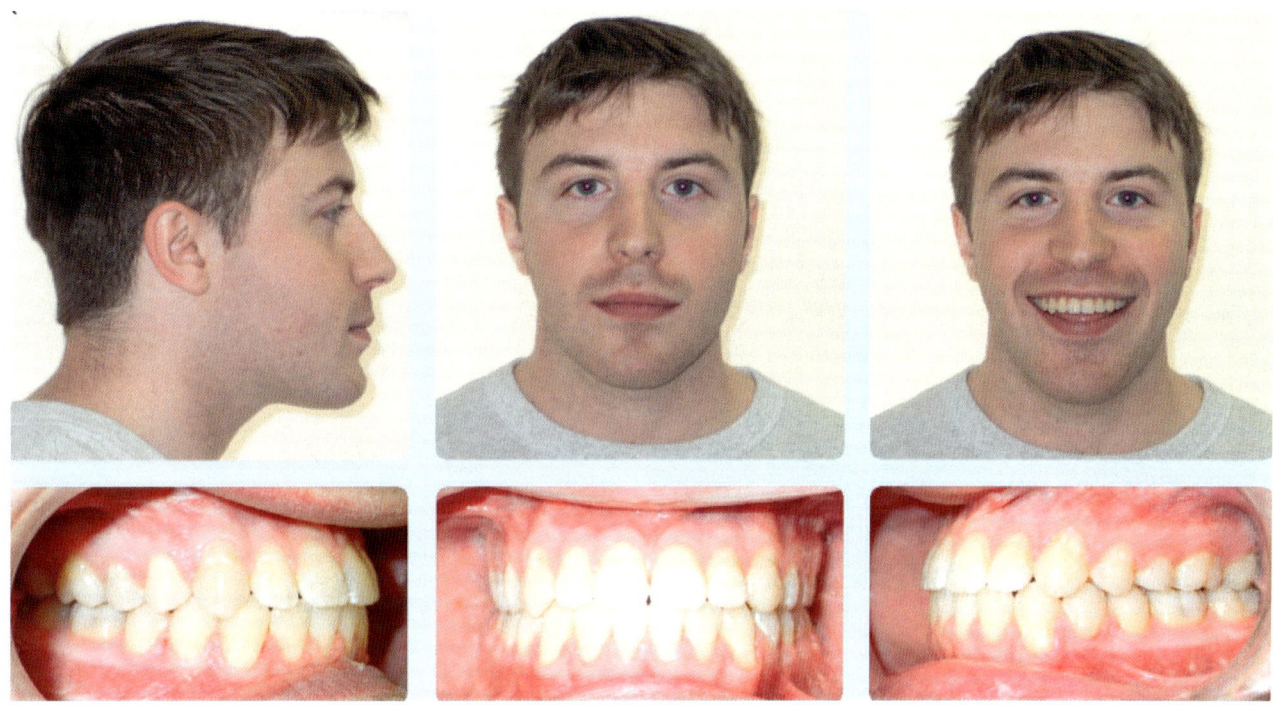

A combined orthodontic and orthognathic surgery approach was taken to correct the bite along with the facial disharmony. Orthognathic surgery was performed by Dr. Derek Steinbacher.

At what age do patients have orthognathic surgery?

Orthognathic surgery is typically performed once a patient is done growing. Those with underbites tend to continue growing later than those with the opposite problem of having excessive overjet. Females tend to stop growing prior to males. The best way to know if growth is complete is to compare cephalometric X-rays from two different points in time. If the size and position of the structures has not changed between the two films, then it's safe to assume growth has finished. The following two X-rays are of the same patient taken at ages sixteen and eighteen. Note how the lower front teeth are more forward in the second X-ray and now are positioned in an underbite. This demonstrates continued growth of the lower jaw.

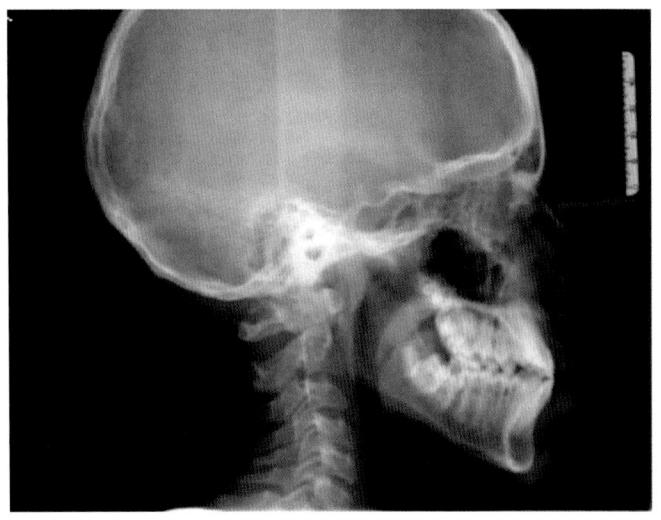
Cephalometric X-ray taken at age sixteen.

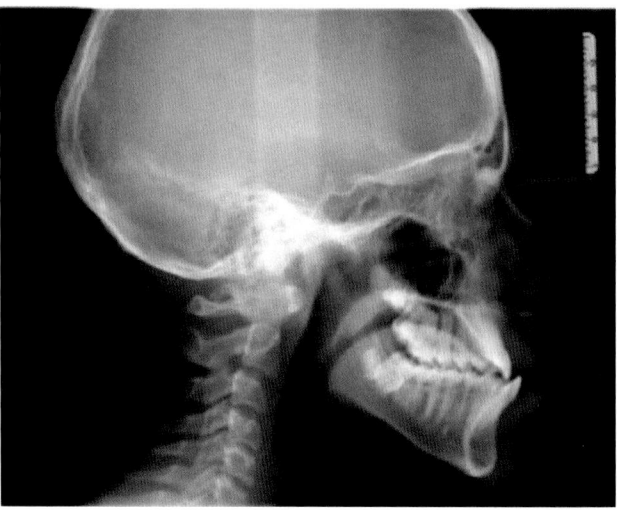
Cephalometric X-ray taken at age eighteen. Note the changes seen in the relative position of the front teeth

7. Retainers

What is a retainer? What types are there? And how long should they be worn for?

A *retainer* is an appliance that aims to hold your teeth in place, and it is the final stage of orthodontic treatment. Some retainers can be glued in, known as *fixed* retainers, while others can come in and out, known as *removable* retainers. Here is an overview of the most common types of retainers:

Essix retainer – An Essix retainer is a clear removable retainer. It is composed of a thin layer of plastic that surrounds and touches all sides of the teeth. This type of retainer looks similar to an aligner and is therefore not very noticeable.

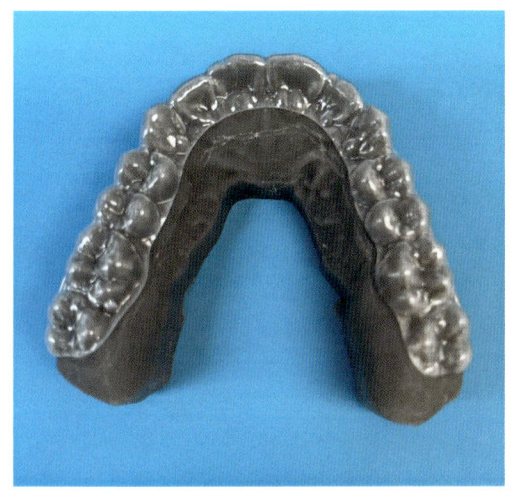

A clear Essix retainer sitting on a model of the teeth.

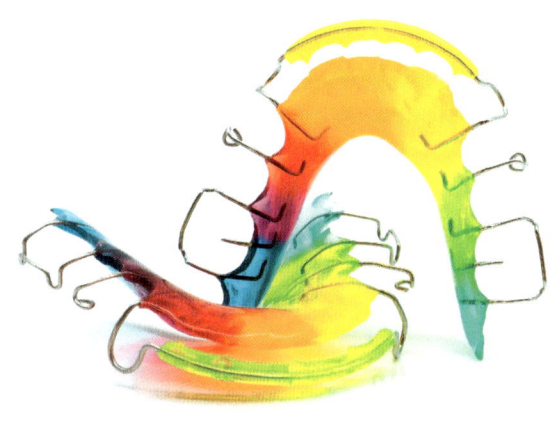

A Hawley retainer

Hawley retainer – This is a more traditional removable retainer made from acrylic and metal wires. Hawley retainers tend to be a little sturdier than Essix retainers. Though they are more noticeable when compared to an Essix, they tend to last longer and are excellent at preventing overbite relapse.

Fixed (permanent) retainer – A permanent retainer involves a metal wire that is bonded behind the teeth. Some patients love this option because one does not have to remember to take it in and out when eating, nor will the retainer ever get lost. A fixed retainer may be a great choice for the child who is always losing their cell phone or forgetting their keys. It is important to maintain good oral hygiene around a permanent retainer, which for some can be challenging. Floss threaders and inter-dental brushes can be used to go underneath the wires to help keep the area clean from plaque and food debris.

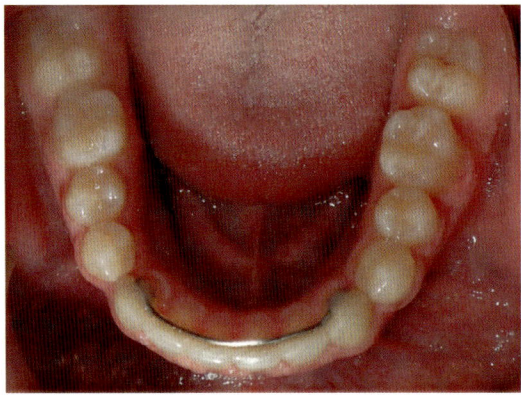 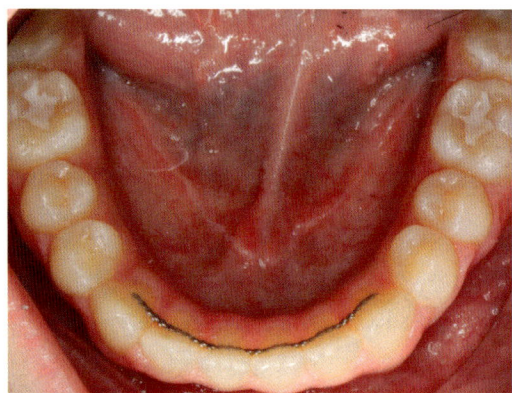

The photos show two different types of permanent retainers. Both are placed from lower canine to lower canine. In the picture on the left, the wire is glued only to the canines, whereas in the picture on the right, the wire is bonded to each of the individual teeth.

Typically, the more you wear the retainer, the more stable the teeth become. Recommendations vary, but on average, we recommend full-time retainer wear (except while eating) for the first three- to six-months after treatment and then only nighttime thereafter.

The orthodontist told my child that they would have to wear their retainer for life! Really?!

You've just spent a lot of time, effort, and money getting your child their ideal smile…you want to keep it that way! Your best shot at maintaining your child's teeth in the same position and preventing *relapse* after completing braces is by wearing a retainer. Their retainer should indeed be worn for the rest of their life. As we age and our bodies change, our teeth continue to move subtly over time. Without a retainer, the teeth may drift back to their original spots prior to starting braces, or even into new undesirable positions. Often when braces are removed, children may feel a relief that the experience is finally over. In reality, keeping their teeth straight is a life-long commitment. Don't let all the hard work that went into their orthodontics be ruined, ensure they are wearing their retainer!

"There is no such thing as good writing, only good rewriting."

– Robert Graves

Creating a work of art is a labor of love. The artist painstakingly agonizes over every stroke of the brush, every word put to paper, and every decision made. Orthodontics gives you the chance to rewrite part of your child's smile story. Perhaps there is a character out of place, the setting isn't quite right, or the finale just didn't come together the way you envisioned. Through guided movement of the teeth and jaws, we can improve the functional and esthetic outcome of your child's smile to craft a more idyllic state. We hope that this chapter provided some important insights into orthodontics, and answered some of the many questions you may have had. So don't be shy. Go snoop around your child's mouth and see if you find any orthodontic concerns.

CHAPTER 10
GENETICS

Have you ever wondered if your dental history and genetics could affect your child's teeth? It's a fascinating topic that has been studied for decades in the field of orthodontics. Relationships undoubtedly exist between parents, children, and siblings for certain dental traits. Understanding these connections can improve treatment recommendations and outcomes. So, let's play a little game of "dental trait detective." Do you still have any baby teeth in your mouth? Were you born missing a permanent tooth? Did you wear an expander or headgear as a kid? Did you have orthognathic surgery in your early twenties? If you have answered "yes" to any of these questions, it's important to let your child's dentist or orthodontist know. This information can help them anticipate any potential issues and provide early intervention if necessary. Embrace your inner detective and let's start investigating those genetic dental traits together!

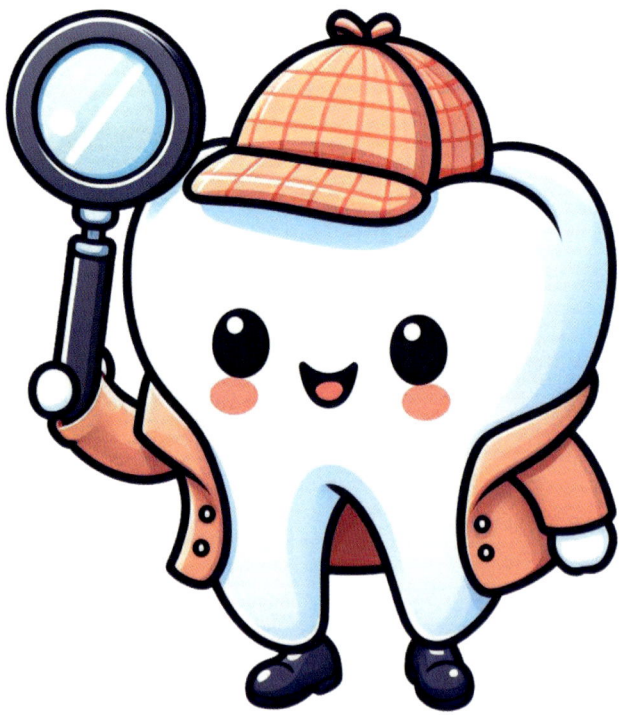

Mandibular Prognathism

One of the most studied genetic traits in orthodontics is the "strong" lower jaw, which can lead to an underbite. If you are a history buff, you may have heard of the infamous "Habsburg Jaw" that persisted through multiple generations of Hungarian and Austrian royalty.[74] The family lineage of such a trait provided a big clue that orofacial structures could be significantly influenced by one's genes. What implication does this have for us today? Well, it's important to remember that individuals with a large lower jaw tend to have a longer growth period. Therefore, if we are suspicious of this genetic tendency, we could use the information to adjust the timing of treatment. We wouldn't want to intervene too soon and have the child outgrow an early intervention (see Chapter 9).

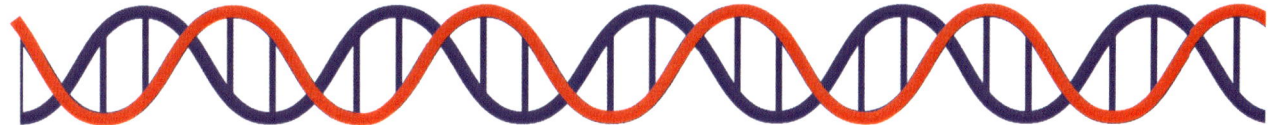

Shorter-than-Average Face

In the previous chapter, we discussed Class 2 malocclusions and noted that their hallmark feature was that the lower teeth were set back relative to the upper teeth. Within the broader group of people that have Class 2 malocclusions, there are a subset of patients with a small lower jaw, a deep bite (100 percent overbite), and upper incisors that tip backwards. These people are referred to as having Class 2 Division 2, and often this is brought about by a shorter-than-average lower part of the face. A study comparing twins and triplets measured the heritable component for this trait and the evidence was overwhelmingly in favor of genetics being the most likely causative factor.[75] These individuals can have significant grinding and clenching problems as a result of their bite. If you have these traits, be on the lookout for signs of bruxism in your child, such as wear or flattening of the back teeth. Though there are other factors that may exacerbate the extent of this type of bite, it is clear that genetics play an underlying role.

Mouth Breathers (with an Open-Bite)

These folks tend to have a longer-than-average face. Often it might be difficult for them to breathe through their nose due to a nasal obstruction issue. While there are various causes of nasal obstruction, genetics has been found to play a role in their development.[76] Here's a simple test to screen your child—sit them down and observe their breathing. If you see that they are breathing through their mouth, ask them to close it and make sure their lips are sealed. Now tell them that they are going to have to keep their lips closed for one whole minute. While their lips are closed, place your finger underneath their nose and check to make sure that air is coming out. If a child has difficulty with this, they will eventually open their mouth and gasp for air. This is a strong indication that they can't breathe easily through their nose, and if that's the case, a visit to your local ENT would be in order.

Congenitally missing teeth or malformed teeth

Missing one or more adult teeth is becoming increasingly common. Up to 9.6 percent of the population is born without a permanent tooth.[77] Fortunately, the most common tooth to be missing is a third molar ("wisdom tooth"). Since most people do not have enough room for their wisdom teeth anyway, being born without them can sometimes be considered a blessing. After the third molar, the next most commonly missing teeth are the lower second premolars and then the upper lateral incisors.[78] If a child is missing teeth, it is important to check their siblings as well, as quite often we will find that this trait runs in families. Depending on the age of the patient, one may not know they are missing until X-rays are taken.

Consider the following example of two sisters. The older sister was born without her upper lateral incisors. This was noticed at a young age, as these teeth failed to appear around their expected eruption time of seven- to eight-years-old. Space was created in these regions for future implants. Naturally, we were on the lookout for missing teeth when her younger sister came in. Upon meeting the younger sister and only having seen photos of her in the past, our initial thought was, "Phew, no missing front teeth." But, after a more thorough investigation, and reviewing the panoramic X-ray, it was evident that though the younger sister lucked out with her front laterals, she was instead missing all four of her second premolars in the back. These teeth are supposed to take the place of the second baby molars (identified by the green arrows). Our plan in this case was to minimize the movement of those teeth in braces and preserve them for as long as possible. By doing so, we improve the prognosis of future implants if and when they are needed.

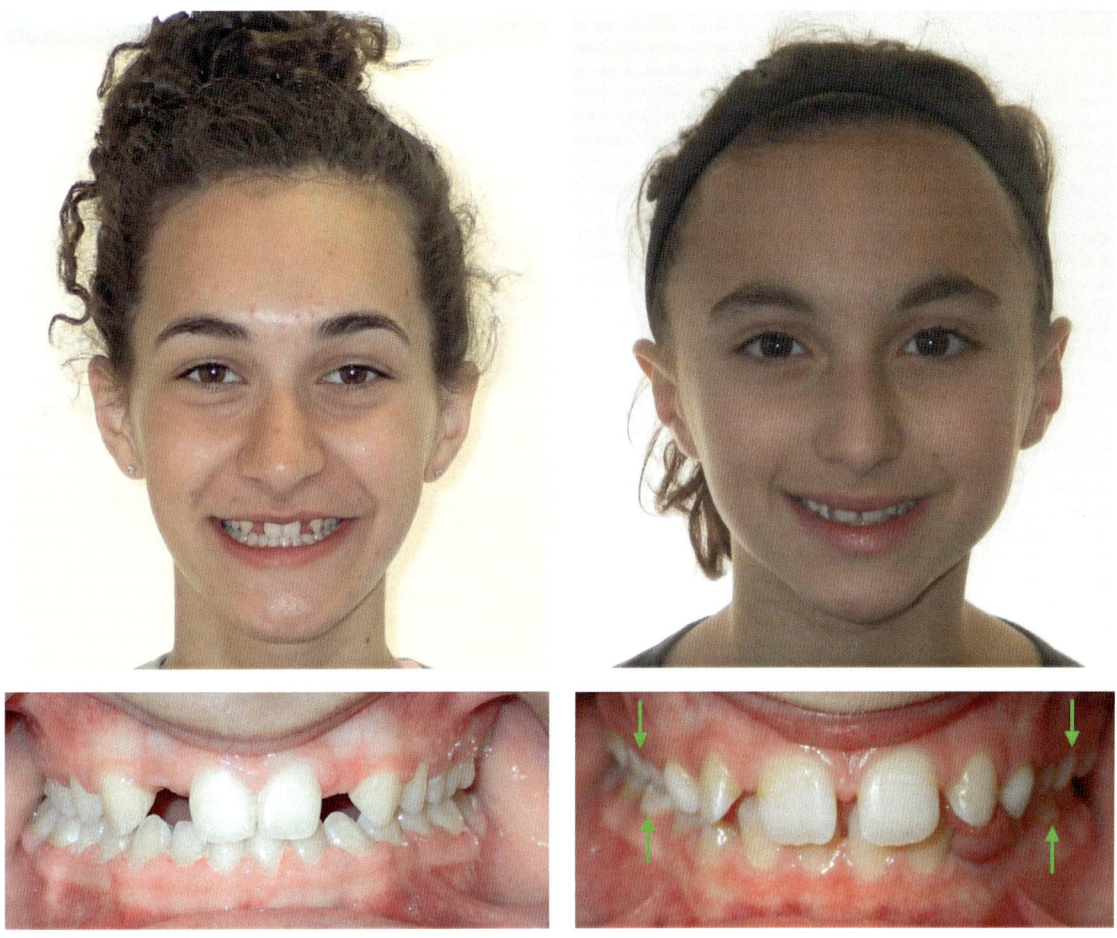

Older sister on the left is born missing upper lateral incisors.
Younger sister on the right is missing four second premolars.

Those who are missing teeth are also more likely to have reduced tooth widths. This sizing anomaly is most commonly seen with the upper lateral incisors, leading to the peg lateral shape that was discussed in Chapter 5. Up to 5 percent of the population has a notable discrepancy in size, which has an effect on the bite and esthetics.[79] By proactively considering the genetic component to these conditions we can get an "early jump" on planning and therapies.

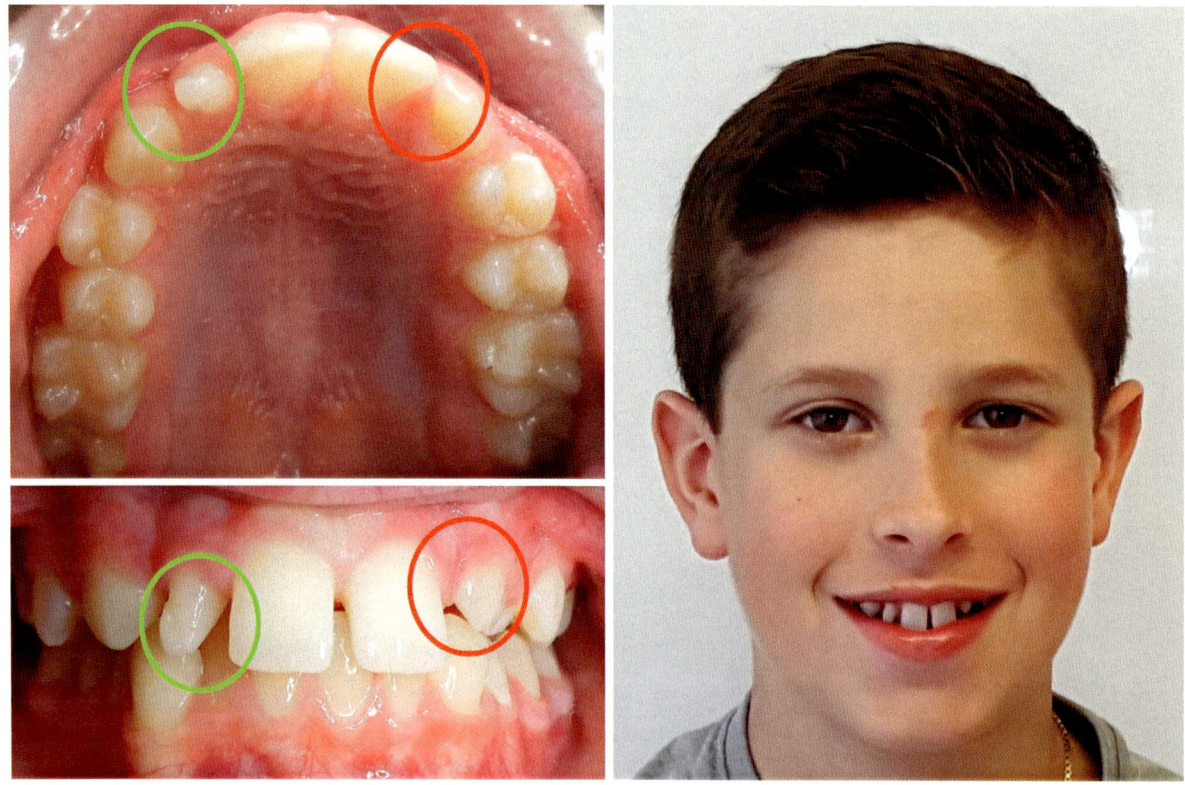

The patient above is missing his upper left lateral incisor. The tooth should be where the red circle currently is. Since he was born without a tooth there, the teeth nearby have shifted in that direction. In addition, the lateral on the other side (green circle) is significantly smaller than it should be; a peg lateral.

Impacted teeth

The incidence of impacted canines in the general population is between 1 and 4 percent.[80] When I am suspicious that a tooth is at risk for impaction, and first bring up the topic with the parent, the response is often: "Oh, I had the same thing as a kid."

"Good to know," I will respond. That information is mighty valuable ahead of time, as kids whose parents had an impacted canine are more likely to have an impacted canine themselves.

Extra teeth

As we discussed in Chapter 5, the most common type of extra tooth is called a mesiodens. This tooth appears in the region of the upper two front teeth and often has unusual anatomy and angulation. Various studies show extra teeth, like the mesiodens, to be more common in boys than girls.[81,82] Though genetic correlation is present, the pattern of inheritance for extra teeth is less clear than the other topics of this chapter. Sometimes extra teeth will be visible in the mouth, but other times, they are only discovered on an X-ray.

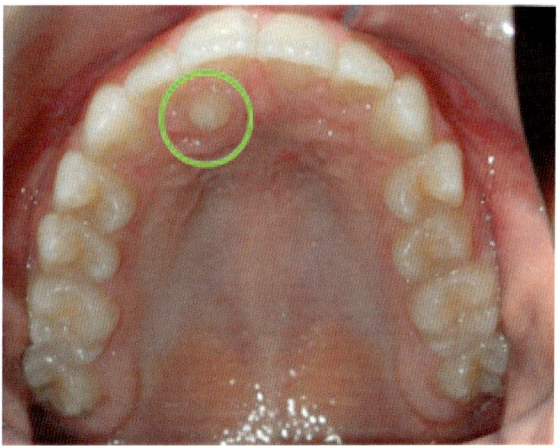

An extra tooth, seen on the roof of the mouth.

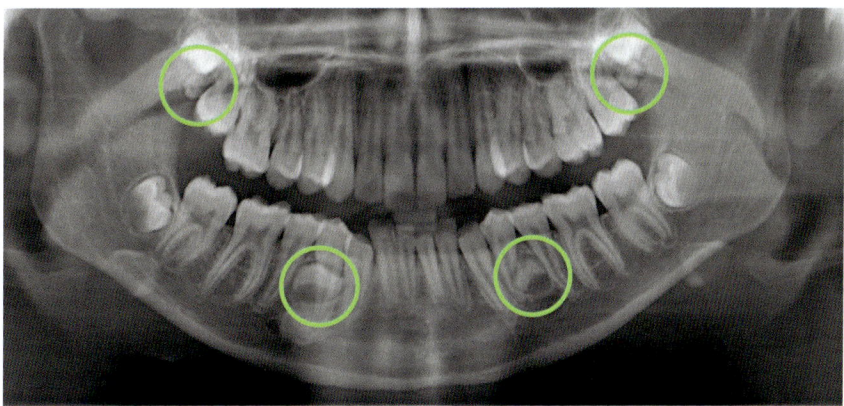

Many extra teeth seen on a panoramic X-ray. Since they are all still developing, this cannot be seen in the mouth without an X-ray.

Periodontitis

Genetics are believed to play a significant role in the development of periodontal disease. Studies have shown that certain individuals are highly susceptible to periodontal disease, while others are more resistant.[83] It is not uncommon to see two patients with similar poor oral hygiene habits, yet one exhibits significant inflammation and bone loss, while the other appears to be generally healthy. There are also differences in how patients respond to periodontal treatment, with some showing marked improvement and others continuing to deteriorate even after multiple rounds of periodontal therapies. Periodontitis tends to run in families, especially the more aggressive forms of the disease.[84] It is therefore recommended to review and be informed of your own dental history and that of your parents. This background can provide insight into the potential likelihood of periodontal disease occurring in your children.

Cavities

Cavities, as we all know by now, are primarily caused by environmental factors such as diet and oral hygiene. However, much like periodontitis, we find that some children are more susceptible than others. Given the same diet and habits, some may suffer from rampant cavities; while others will be less affected. There is growing data to show that genetics play a role in the development of cavities. In particular, factors that relate to the development of enamel, saliva strength, and immune response are believed to have a genetic component to them.[85]

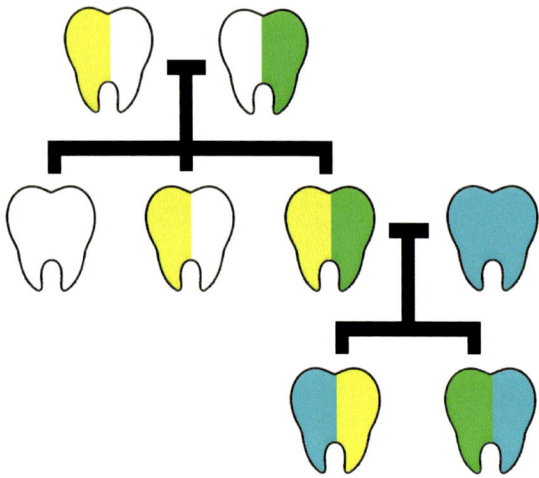

> **"Mystery creates wonder and wonder is the basis of man's desire to understand."**
>
> **– Neil Armstrong**

Hopefully that detective hat was on tight as we investigated the mysteries of your child's smile. Our oral health is truly the product of both nature and nurture. While we cultivate a beautiful smile through love and care, there are genetic forces at play that should not be discounted. Understanding the relative influence of each can help clinicians and parents know what to expect and how best to tailor treatment.

CHAPTER 11
GUM HEALTH

Would you want to build your home atop shifting sands or a boggy swamp? Of course not! Any architect in their right mind would only start construction on solid ground. Healthy gums are the literal foundation upon which our smiles are built. They surround, stabilize, and attach the teeth to the bone underneath. Take care of the gums and they will provide you a lifetime of sturdy support; neglect them, and the whole base collapses out from under you. The consequences of gum disease can be severe with a tremendous drop off in the quality of one's life. Pain, tooth loss, cardiovascular disease, diabetes, pregnancy complications, Alzheimer's disease…the list of conditions associated with gum disease is a veritable A-to-Z of maladies you'll want to avoid. In this section, we hope to make you the architect of a bright future for your child's smile by impressing upon you the importance of healthy gums.

How do I tell the difference between healthy and unhealthy gums?

In order to recognize disease, we must first know what normal looks like. Pink is the name of the game when it comes to healthy gums. The gums, which are technically called the *gingiva*, are typically light pink, stippled in texture (similar to an orange peel), and firm against the teeth. As discussed in Chapter 7, there should not be any bleeding when brushing or flossing. On the other hand, unhealthy gums usually appear a bright angry red, lose their stippling, and can be described as "puffy." Plaque and tartar are often present, and bleeding can occur when performing oral hygiene. In severe cases, the gums may be so fragile that bleeding can happen just by chewing, or worse yet, be spontaneous without any provocation at all. So, let's try to avoid "seeing red" and aim to "think pink."

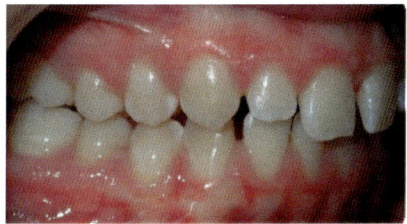 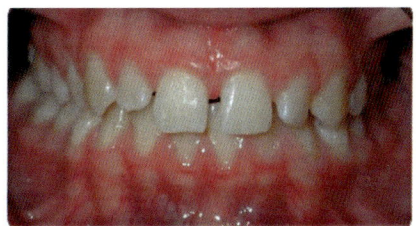 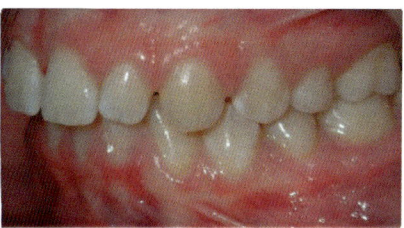

Healthy – Twelve-year-old with minimal inflammation and healthy gums.

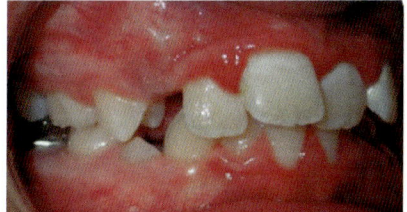 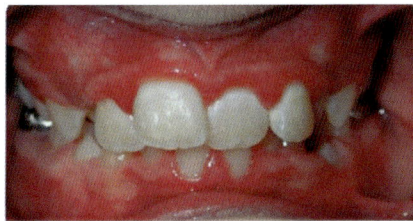 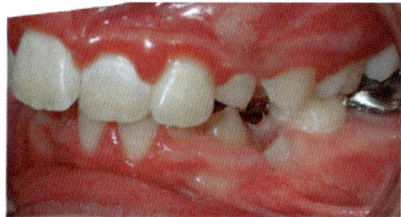

Unhealthy – Ten-year-old with inflamed gums and evidence of plaque.

Remind me…what causes gingivitis?

Gingivitis is one of the most common conditions of the mouth and it frequently occurs in children. The culprit? Bacteria from plaque that sticks to the tooth surface and invades the gum tissue leading to inflammation. Fortunately, because this inflammation is due in large part to poor oral hygiene, it is often preventable and correctable with proper oral care.

What is the difference between plaque and tartar?

While plaque is a mushy mixture of bacteria and food debris, *tartar*, or what dentists refer to as *calculus*, is a solidified deposit. You can think of the difference between plaque and tartar as akin to the difference between wet cement and hardened concrete. Over time, minerals such as calcium and phosphate, which occur naturally in our saliva, are absorbed by the plaque, causing it to set and transform into the hardened mass of tartar. This hardening process is gradual, so the presence of tartar generally indicates that oral hygiene has not been performed well enough over an extended period of time. Another significant difference is that tartar is extremely difficult to remove by brushing and flossing alone. Instead, it must be physically dislodged by dental professionals in order to remove it completely.

What is periodontitis? What makes it so significantly worse than gingivitis?

Here's a question for you...why do you think most adults lose their teeth? Your first instinct might be to say, "it's because of tooth decay." But the truth is that when children grow up, most will actually lose their teeth due to the gum disease known as *periodontitis*.[86]

Throughout this book, we have discussed the topic of gingivitis—its cause, appearance, and treatment. Now imagine if gingivitis went unchecked; like any disease, the condition would only become more rampant and destructive. While the inflammation of gingivitis is limited to the surface layers of gum tissue, the destruction in periodontitis goes deeper, destroying the underlying bone that supports the teeth and holds them in place. This is bad news! With enough bone loss, the adult teeth may start to become loose and may eventually fall out. Sounds bad right? Well just you wait...it gets worse! Because the bone loss associated with periodontitis is *irreversible*. The body has a very difficult time building new bone around the teeth. At these later stages of the disease, no amount of improved hygiene can restore what was lost.

We tend to think of periodontitis as a disease of adults and the elderly, but make no mistake, children can get periodontitis too! All it takes is the right combination of bacteria and neglect. Regular dental visits are highly recommended to make sure that periodontal disease, if present, is treated in its early stages when treatment is most predictable.[87, 88]

What is a periodontal "pocket" and why is it important?

A *periodontal pocket* is a thin gap between each tooth and its surrounding gum tissue. Just like how lint can accumulate in the bottom of clothing pockets, so too can bacteria and food debris collect and hide out in the base of these biologic pockets. In healthy, non-inflamed gums, they should be very shallow (less than four-millimeters). So long as the pocket is shallow, normal brushing and flossing can clean it out thoroughly, but if the pocket is too deep (over five-millimeters), plaque and tartar can become sheltered in its depths, inaccessible to routine home care. If the child is unable to clean the pocket fully, the presence of longstanding bacterial contamination will contribute to continued destruction of the supporting structures of the teeth, further deepening the pocket and leading to eventual tooth loss.

What is the difference between a deep cleaning and a regular dental cleaning?

The main difference between a "regular" and "deep" cleaning is the extensiveness of the procedure. A regular cleaning, typically done twice per year, involves removing superficial plaque and tartar deposits while polishing the teeth to make them nice and shiny. This type of cleaning is done when the gums are healthy and only routine maintenance is required. A deep cleaning, or what dentists call *scaling and root planing*, is performed when the gums are in a diseased state. The deep cleaning is focused more at debriding below the gum line, on the root surface of the tooth. This procedure becomes necessary if the patient has the aforementioned deep periodontal pockets, where plaque and tartar are otherwise out of reach. Unlike a regular cleaning, this procedure is usually performed with local anesthesia to numb the area and minimize discomfort as the dentist or hygienist physically scrapes away the bacterial deposits. After the deep cleaning is performed, there will be an approximately four– to six-week healing period, at which point a reassessment will be done to check the pockets and see whether any further treatment is necessary.

My child has inflamed gums, but their hygiene seems pretty good. What am I missing?

In addition to poor oral hygiene, there are a few other factors that can exaggerate our body's response to dental plaque. The first is the onset of puberty. As discussed in our chapter on early adolescence, the hormonal changes occurring at that time skew our body's responsiveness to plaque, worsening the inflammation seen. If your daughter has just recently started menstruating and her gums have become puffier, this is a likely explanation. Another modifying factor is the use of certain prescription medications. These include anti-seizure medications, calcium channel blockers (used to treat hypertension), and immunosuppressants.[89,90] These drugs can lead to significant overgrowth of the gingiva, known as *hypertrophy*, causing it to appear very large and bulbous. When the growth is due to medications, you and your child's physician will need to weigh the gum issue against the importance of staying on the medication to maintain their overall health. Switching to an alternative prescription drug may be an option in some cases.

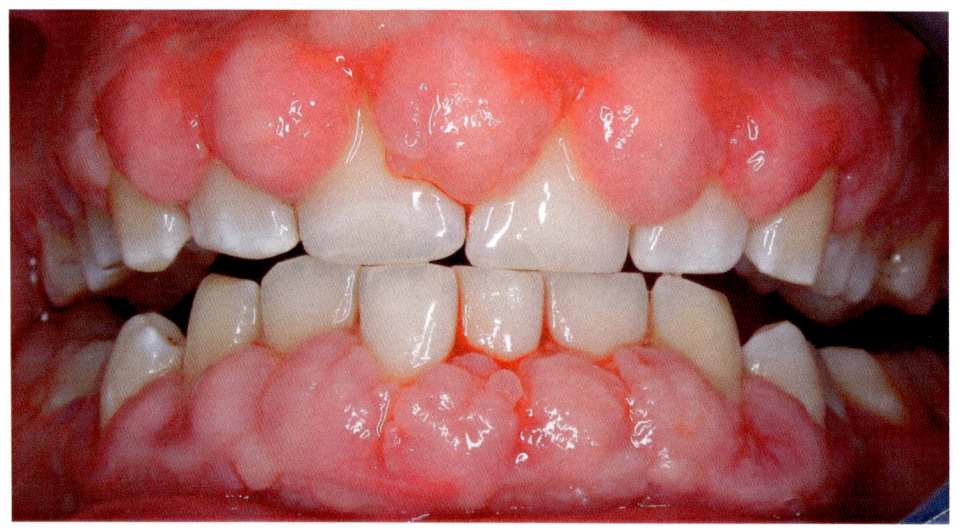
An example of gingival hypertrophy

What does an abscess look like on the gums?

Abscesses are contained areas of *pus*, a thick yellow/white fluid made up of dead cells and bacteria. In the gums, this pus may originate from an infected tooth or from a periodontal pocket. The abscess will appear as a dome shaped bubble on the gums. It may be pink like the surrounding gingiva, a brighter red, or have a yellowish tint due to the pus contained within. As the pus continues to build, sometimes the bubble bursts, spewing the goop out and leaving the child with a foul taste in their mouth. Other times the pressure can cause the pus to spread to other parts of the body, resulting in serious bouts of swelling and systemic infection. Treatment options for abscesses can entail either a root canal, gum surgery, or extraction depending on the cause and extent of the infection. An abscess is not something to be trifled with. If you notice one, get treatment as soon as possible.

What if there's a bubble on the lips, is that an abscess?

Unlikely. An abscess will be in close proximity to the tooth it is associated with. If there is a bubble on the lip, especially the lower lip, the more probable explanation is something known as a *mucocele*. Mucoceles are painless, fluid-filled blisters that are most common in childhood. They are usually brought on when children accidentally bite their lips or cheeks. It usually goes unnoticed, but our bodies are always producing saliva. The saliva is made in glands and transported to the mouth through a network of tiny structures called *ducts*. When a child bites their lip, they may inadvertently sever one of these

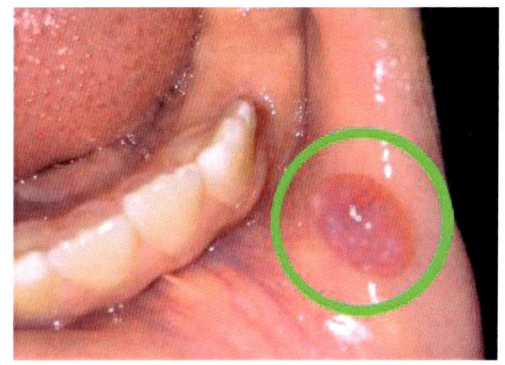

A mucocele seen on the right portion of the lower lip.

salivary ducts. You can think of ducts like the plumbing system in your kitchen. If a pipe bursts, all the water will start spilling out under your sink, and similarly, if the duct bursts, it's the saliva that spills out into the lip and pools beneath the surface. Most mucoceles will resolve on their own, but for larger bubbles, or those that continue to be traumatized, they may need to be surgically removed.

What is gum recession?

Gum recession is the migration of gingival tissue further down the root of a tooth.[91] When roots are exposed, significant sensitivity may occur. Unlike enamel, the root surface will fire off pain signals in response to hot and cold temperatures. If severe, you may even have to say "goodbye" to enjoying your favorite ice cream or specialty coffee! There is also a higher risk of cavity formation on the softer, exposed root surface as compared to the hard enamel of the crown. Additionally, gum recession presents a serious esthetic concern for most patients. Would you want to smile with your roots showing? We don't think so. If your dentist suspects that recession is developing, they may refer you to a periodontist (a gum specialist) for monitoring or treatment.

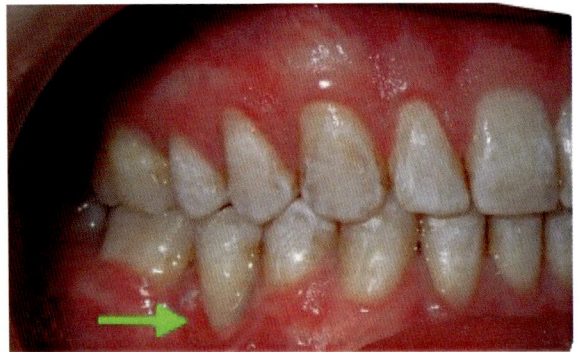 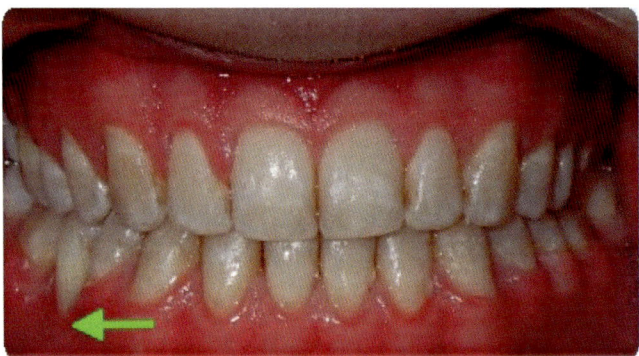

Gum recession seen on a single tooth (green arrow).

What is the treatment for recession?

Unfortunately, once your gums have migrated down onto the root, they cannot grow back on their own. Let this be just another reminder of how important prevention is. The only option to correct the problem is surgery. *Soft tissue grafts* are the treatment of choice for gum recession. The graft is a patch of tissue that must first be harvested, usually from the roof of the patient's mouth. In certain situations, donor tissue may be utilized. It is then stitched in place to cover the exposed roots and restore the esthetic appearance of the gums. While our roots may be very hard workers, they do not crave the spotlight, so let's keep them working behind the scenes where they belong.

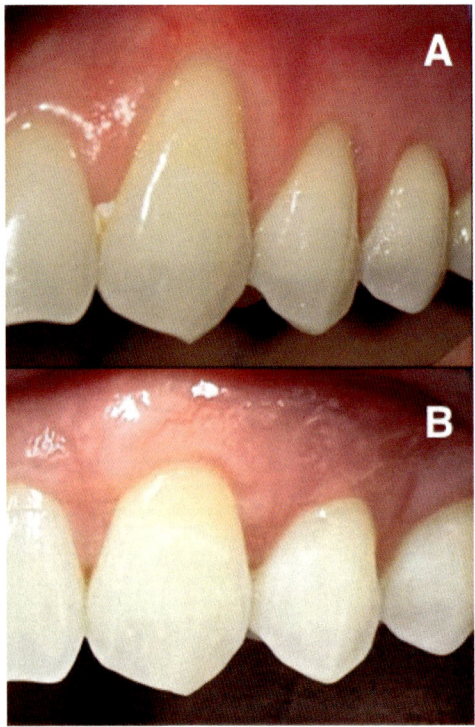

In (A), recession is seen on the patient's canine. (B) shows the same patient's gums twelve-weeks after receiving a graft.

What if my child's gums are more dark (brownish) than pink?

Do not worry, just like our eyes, hair, and skin, there is significant variation in "normal" gingival color. Some children are simply born with areas of darker pigmentation than others. These kids tend to have more *melanin* in their gums. Melanin is the pigment that helps protect us from the sun's UV rays. Darker gingiva is most common in African and Mediterranean populations, but can occur in those with lighter skin tones as well. Usually, the pigmentation remains stable over time. This consistency of appearance is an important distinction. If you do notice new spots, spots that have been growing in size, or spots with significantly different colors or irregular borders, you should discuss them with a healthcare professional to see if any follow up or treatment is indicated.

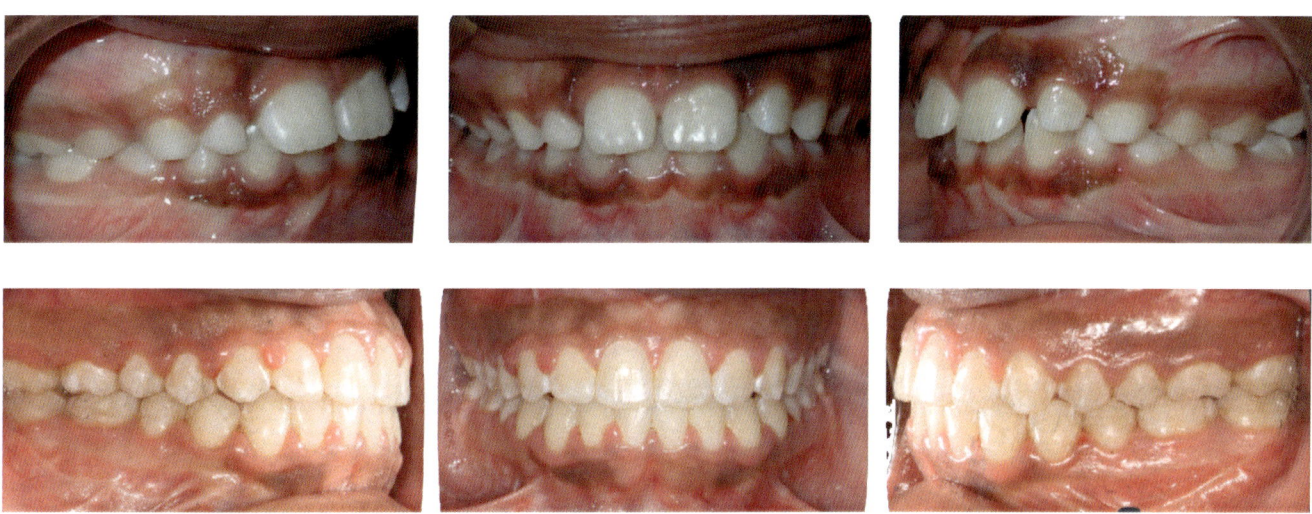

Two examples of pigmentation of the gum tissue. Note the high degree of variation that is possible.

What is a frenum and how can it impact the teeth and gums?

A frenum is a band or flap of soft tissue that appears like a muscle attachment inside the mouth connecting different oral structures. While there are several frenums in the mouth, the ones that get the most attention are typically the labial frenum, located between the upper front two teeth, and the lingual frenum, which is associated with tongue-ties. A frenum that is large or attached irregularly is a risk factor for causing gum recession. It may also impact the spacing between the teeth, causing gaps to open up in response to the strong muscle pull. Tight frenum attachments may impact speech or a baby's ability to breastfeed (see our discussion of ankyloglossia in Chapter 3). Depending on the extent of the frenum, your dentist or orthodontist may suggest that it be trimmed. The timing of this procedure is determined on a case-by-case basis. Sometimes this is done at an early age, and sometimes it's performed around the time a child is undergoing orthodontic treatment.

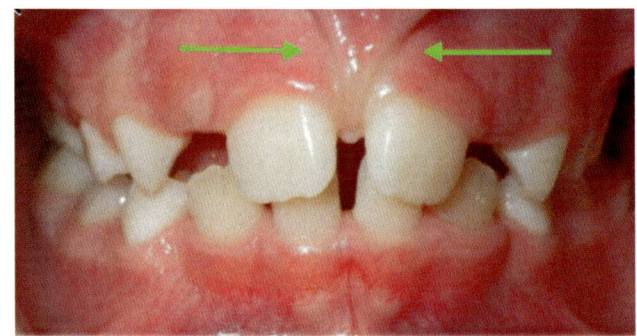

Labial frenum seen between the two front teeth. Depending on the size and position, it can lead to a space between the two front teeth.

What is the relationship between gum health and overall well-being?

Poor gum health can be a harbinger of a plethora of systemic conditions and disorders, including diabetes, cardiovascular diseases, Alzheimer's disease, obesity, and inflammatory bowel disease. For example, pathogenic oral bacteria have been identified in atherosclerotic plaques in the circulatory system. The bacteria in the mouth induce a local inflammatory response in the gums, which prompts the production of *cytokines* (signaling proteins) which enter the bloodstream and trigger a cascade of events leading to a chronic inflammatory state.[92] Although the human body is resilient, let's always remember that everything is interconnected, and what happens in the mouth can affect the rest of the body as well.

"The best way to find yourself is to lose yourself in the service of others."

– Mahatma Gandhi

Our gums find their purpose in the support and service of our smile. While our teeth may be the stars of the show, the truth is that a beautiful smile is really the result of a full cast of characters working together. The roots, gingiva, and bones of the jaw all have their parts to play in this diverse ensemble performance. Don't overlook their contributions to our oral health—take care of them and they will take care of you.

CHAPTER 12
AIRWAY AND SLEEP

Welcome to the chapter that discusses the connection between the airway, sleep, and teeth! You may be wondering why we've dedicated a section of our book specifically to this topic. Well, how we breathe profoundly impacts the growth of our facial bones, directly influencing the beauty of our smiles and the alignment of our bite. Sleep is a precious time for both body and mind to rest and regenerate. As parents, you know firsthand how a single night of poor sleep can disrupt your entire day. Now imagine the long-term effects your child may experience if they consistently struggle with sleep. Although the link may not be immediately obvious, we encourage you to join us in exploring this final chapter and know that the knowledge you gain here will have a lasting positive impact on your child.

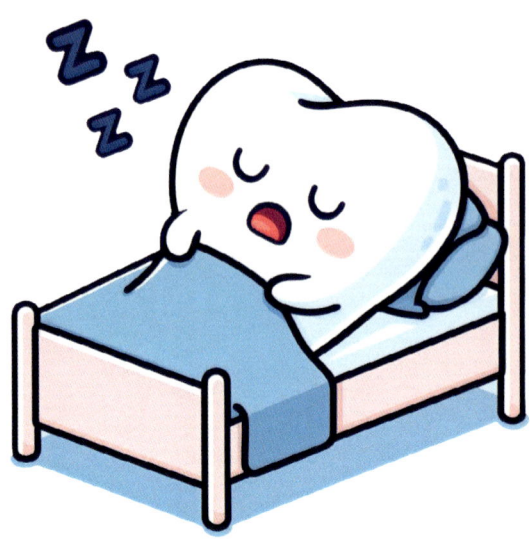

I have noticed that my child is snoring. At what point should I be concerned?

It might be tempting to believe that the loud sounds coming from your child's bedroom at night are a definitive sign of a breathing or sleeping issue, but perhaps surprisingly, snoring alone is not always a problem. Our true concern is that snoring might be a sign of a condition called obstructive sleep apnea (OSA).

What is Obstructive Sleep Apnea (OSA)?

Obstructive sleep apnea (OSA) occurs when the upper airway becomes partially or completely blocked during sleep. This leads to pauses in breathing, interruptions in the flow of oxygen to the lungs, and fragmented sleep.[93] Obstructive sleep apnea is associated with various issues related to inadequate high-quality sleep, such as behavioral problems, difficulties with concentration and focus, and impaired school performance. OSA affects approximately twenty-five million people in the United States and is a common form of sleep-disordered breathing.[94]

How do I know if my child has OSA?

Obstructive sleep apnea is accompanied by a range of signs and symptoms that can lead to such a diagnosis. The most notable indicators are snoring, restless sleep, morning fatigue, and quick sleep onset. Other findings include hyperactivity, bed-wetting, and poor behavior. Sometimes it can be difficult to know if a child is experiencing OSA versus another behavioral issue (like ADHD), and in such cases, your pediatrician may recommend a *sleep study* to help find the answer. This is usually performed overnight in a hospital or sleep facility, but some home studies are available with varying degrees of accuracy.

What should I do if I suspect OSA?

First, discuss your concerns with your child's primary care provider. They are likely to refer you to a sleep specialist or a pediatric otolaryngologist (ENT). They will review the signs and symptoms and perform an examination to determine if further testing is required.

I have noticed that my child sleeps with their mouth open and is always thirsty in the morning. What does that mean?

This probably means that the child has some degree of upper airway obstruction. The *tonsils and/or adenoids* are a frequent culprit for this obstruction, but there are other causes to be considered as well.[95] It may also be a sign of OSA. Frequent mouth breathing can have long-lasting effects on growth as was discussed in Chapter 9 on orthodontics. An evaluation with a pediatrician or an ENT is likely in order.

What are the tonsils and adenoids? What purpose do they serve?

The *tonsils* are a collection of paired lymphoid tissues located throughout our upper airway. One set of these tonsils is known as the *adenoids*. In fact, the technical term for the adenoids is the *pharyngeal tonsils*, named after their location in the pharynx. Without the aid of specialized instruments, the adenoids are not visible when looking into your child's mouth or nose. Instead, when you look into the mouth of a child, and have them say "Ahhhh," you may be able to visualize their *palatine tonsils*, located behind their tongue. The lymph tissues that make up our tonsils play a role in helping the body fight infections.

Why should tonsils and adenoids be removed if they help fight infections?

Sometimes these structures get too large, leading to obstructed breathing. This can result in obstructive sleep apnea or irregular dental and facial growth patterns as mentioned earlier. Additionally, enlarged adenoids can harbor a reservoir of bacteria, causing recurrent upper respiratory infections and contributing to ear infections or fluid accumulation.

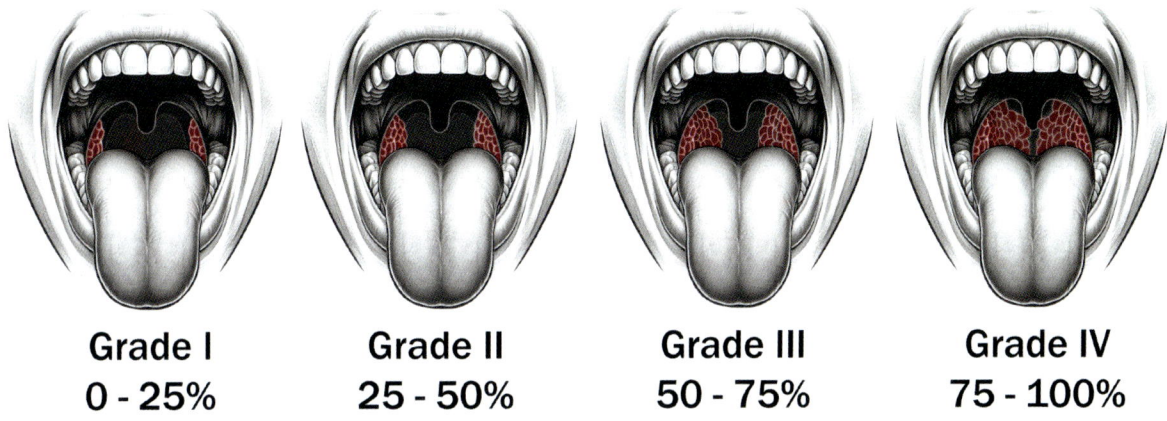

Enlarged tonsils may block the airway and lead to OSA.

Why might an ENT suggest removing only the adenoids, while leaving the tonsils?

The recovery process from a tonsillectomy (surgically removing the palatine tonsils from the back of the throat) is considerably more challenging compared to an adenoidectomy alone. The ENT can assess the primary cause of your child's symptoms. If the symptoms are mainly attributed to the adenoids, and the tonsils are not significantly contributing to the problem, it is typically not recommended to remove them. This will spare the child the difficult post-surgery period from having their tonsils out.

Can I wait to get my child's tonsils out?

The answer is "maybe." This depends on why they need to be removed and what cause there might be for waiting. If the reason for removal is infection or obstructive sleep apnea, it is important to remember that these symptoms will probably persist until the problem is addressed. If you feel that there is a good reason to wait, then it is important to understand the risks and to review them with your child's ENT doctor.

How does nasal obstruction affect my child's teeth?

Nasal obstruction can affect the teeth in two main ways. Firstly, nasal obstruction forces children to breathe through their mouth more, and mouth breathing tends to lead to oral dryness, increasing the risk of dental cavities. Saliva plays a protective role for teeth, and its reduction, therefore, can be problematic. Secondly, chronic mouth breathing can alter dental facial growth, causing the lower jaw to grow more downwards, creating a high-arched narrow palate and dental crowding. This frequently requires orthodontic treatment to correct.

"A good laugh and a long sleep are the best cures in the doctor's book."

– Irish Proverb

Perhaps the narrative of your child's smile has always been a bedtime story. Hopefully it's a peaceful tale of rest and relaxation, but if it's plagued by tossing and turning, do not hesitate to seek help. The value of a good night's sleep cannot be overstated.

CONCLUSION

We hope you enjoyed our dental journey together. At a minimum, you are much more aware of your child's oral health, and likely your own too. At a maximum, you are switching careers and becoming a dentist! Either way, by taking the time to read this book, your child's mouth is likely better off because of it. Remember to prioritize visits to the dentist for preventative care and make oral hygiene an important part of your child's daily routine. We wish you and your child a lifetime of healthy smiles!

The QR code on the following page sends you to a list of the authors' favorite products. Check them out!

THE TOOTH BIBLE'S SMILE SHOP WITH OUR RECOMMENDED PRODUCT LIST

TheToothBible.com

Helpful Links:

- American Cleft Lip and Palate – Find a Team
    https://acpacares.org/find-a-care-team

- CDC My Water's Fluoride
    https://nccd.cdc.gov/doh_mwf/default/default.aspx

- Radiology Dose Calculator
    https://www.ans.org/nuclear/dosechart/

- USDA Dietary Recommendations
    https://www.myplate.gov/eat-healthy/what-is-myplate

Photo Acknowledgments:

Page 4: From left to right (Eleven years, Nine years, Seven years), courtesy of Catherine King Photography

Page 6: Wedding photo, courtesy of Katie Slater Photography

Page 32: 5-year-old twins, courtesy of Catherine Kiernan Photography

Page 115: Allure Mini Bracket, courtesy of Allure Ortho

Page 115: Essence Bracket, courtesy of Allure Ortho

Page 116: Experience Self-ligating Brackets, courtesy of GC Orthodontics

Page 128: Inbrace Lingual Braces, courtesy of Inbrace

Page 139: Two types of retainers, courtesy of Dr. Eric Frank, Oceans Orthodontics and Pediatric Dentistry

REFERENCES

1. Cate Ten AR. *Oral Histology: Development, structure, and function.* 5th ed. Mosby, 1998.

2. Profitt WR, Fields Jr HW, Server DM. *Contemporary Orthodontics.* 5th ed. Mosby, 2013.

3. Caufield PW, Li Y, Bromage TG. Hypoplasia-associated severe early childhood caries–A proposed definition. *J Dent Res* 91, no.6 (2012): 544-50.

4. Offenbacher S, Katz V, Fertik G, et al. Periodontal infection as a possible risk factor for preterm low birth weight. *J Periodontology* 67, no.105 (1996): 1103-1113.

5. Dasanayake AP. Poor periodontal health of the pregnant woman as a risk factor for low birth weight. *Annals of Periodontology* 3, no.1 (1998): 206-212.

6. Lopez, NJ, Smith PC, Gutierrez. Periodontal Therapy May Reduce the Risk of Preterm Low Birth Weight in Women with Periodontal Disease: A Randomized Controlled Trial. *J Periodontolgy* 73, no.8 (2002): 911-924.

7. Dixon, MJ, Marazita ML, Beaty TH, Murray JC. Cleft Lip and Palate: Understanding genetic and environmental influences. *Nat Rev Genet* 12, no.3 (2011): 167-178

8. American Academy of Pediatric Dentistry. Periodicity of examination, preventive dental services, anticipatory guidance/counseling, and oral treatment for infants, children, and adolescents. *The Reference Manual of Pediatric Dentistry.* Chicago, Ill.: American Academy of Pediatric Dentistry; 2021:241-51.

9. Davey AL, Rogers AH. Multiple types of the bacterium Streptococcus mutans in the human mouth and their intra-family transmission. *Arch Oral Biol* 29, no.6 (1984): 453-60.

10. New York State Department of Health. Oral health care during pregnancy and early childhood: Practice Guidelines. August 2006.

11. CDC. Recommendations for using fluoride to prevent and control dental caries in the United States. MMWR Recomm Rep 2001;50(RR-14):1-42

12. McDonagh MS, Whiting PF, Bradley M, et al. A Systematic Review of Public Water Fluoridation. University of York, York: NHS Centre for Reviews and Dissemination, September 2000. Community Preventive Services Task Force. Guide to Community Preventive Services: Preventing Dental Caries: Community Water Fluoridation website.

13. MMWR. Morbidity and mortality weekly report, Vol. 70, no. 21 Corporate Authors(s): Centers for Disease Control and Prevention (U.S.) Published Date: 05/28/2021

14. American Academy of Pediatric Dentistry. Fluoride therapy. *The Reference Manual of Pediatric Dentistry.* Chicago, IL: American Academy of Pediatric Dentistry, (2023): 352-8.

15. American Academy of Pediatrics: Poison treatment in the home. American Academy of Pediatrics Committee on Injury, Violence and Poison Prevention, Pediatrics 112:1182-1185, 2003.

16. Tham R, Bowatte G, Dharmage SC, et al. Breastfeeding and the risk of dental caries: A systematic review and meta-analysis. *Acta Paediatr* 104, no.467 (2015): 62-84.

17. American Academy of Pediatric Dentistry. Policy on early childhood caries (ECC): Consequences and preventive strategies. *The Reference Manual of Pediatric Dentistry*. Chicago, Ill.: American Academy of Pediatric Dentistry; 2021:81-4.

18. Heyman MB, Abrams SA. AAP Section On Gastroenterology, Hepatology, And Nutrition, AAP Committee On Nutrition. Fruit Juice in Infants, Children, and Adolescents: Current Recommendations. *Pediatrics* 139, no.6 (2017)

19. Otto M, "How can a child die of a toothache in the US?" *The Guardian*. June 13, 2017. http://www.theguardian.com/inequality/2017/jun/13/healthcare-gap-how-can-a-child-die-of-toothache-in-the-us

20. John J, Weddell JA, Shin DE, Jones JJ. Gingivitis and periodontal disease. In: JA Dean, ed. McDonald and Avery's Dentistry for the Child and Adolescent, 10th ed. Maryland Heights, Mo.: Mosby Elsevier; 2016:243-73.

21. Segal L, Stephenson R, Dawes M, Feldman P. Prevalence, diagnosis, and treatment of ankyloglossia. *Can Fam Physician* 53, no.6 (2007):1027-33.

22. Boutsi EZ, Tatakis DN. Maxillary labial frenum attachment in children. *Int J Paediatr Dent* 21 no.4 (2011):284-8.16. Schmitt DL, Johnson DW, Henderson FW. Herpes simplex type 1 infections in group day care. *Pediatr Infect Dis J* 10, no.10 (1991): 729-34.

23. Schmitt DL, Johnson DW, Henderson FW. Herpes simplex type 1 infections in group day care. *Pediatr Infect Dis J* 10, no.10 (1991): 729-34.

24. Amir J. Clinical aspects and antiviral therapy in primary herpetic gingivostomatitis. *Paediatr Drugs* 3, no.8 (2001): 593-7.

25. American Academy of Pediatrics. Herpes simplex. In: Red Book: 2021-2024 Report of the Committee on Infectious Diseases, 32nd ed, Kimberlin DW, Barnett ED, Lynfield R, Sawyer MH (Eds), American Academy of Pediatrics, Itasca, IL 2021. p.407.

26. Whittington BR, Durward CS. Survey of anomalies in primary teeth and their correlation with the permanent dentition. *NZ Dent J* 92, no. 407 (1996): 4-8.

27. American Nuclear Society. "Radiation Dose Calculator – ANS / About Nuclear." Accessed November 30, 2023. https://www.ans.org/nuclear/dosechart

28. American Academy of Pediatric Dentistry. Policy on use of fluoride. *The Reference Manual of Pediatric Dentistry*. Chicago, Ill.: American Academy of Pediatric Dentistry; (2023): 100-2.

29. Hartman NR, Mao JJ, Zhou H, Boyne MT, Wasserman AM, Taylor K, Racoosin JA, Patel V, Colatsky T. More methemoglobin is produced by benzocaine treatment than lidocaine treatment in human in vitro systems. *Regul Toxicol Pharmacol* 70, (2014): 182-8.

30. Mehta V, Singh RK. Congenitally missing primary and permanent maxillary lateral incisors. *BMJ Case Rep*. Oct 7 (2016) doi: 10.1136/bcr-2016-216779.

31. Centers for Disease Control and Prevention. Vital signs: dental sealant use and untreated tooth decay among US school-aged children. *MMWR* 65, no.41 (2016):1141-1145.

32. Centers for Disease Control and Prevention. "Dental Sealants Prevent Cavities." Accessed Nov 30, 2023. https://www.cdc.gov/vitalsigns/pdf/2016-10-vitalsigns.pdf

33. TP-CERHR Monograph on the Potential human reproductive and development effects of bisphenol A. National Toxicology Program, U.S. Department of Health and Human Services. National Institutes of Health. NIH Publication No. 08-5994.2008.

34. Fleisch AF, Sheffield PE, Chinn C, Edelstein BL, Landrigan PJ. Bisphenol A and related compounds in dental materials. *Pediatrics* 126, no.4 (2012): 760-8.

35. Joskow R, Barr DB, Barr JR, et al. Exposure to bisphenol A from bis-glycidyl dimethacrylate-based dental sealants. *J Am Dent Assoc* 137, no.3 (2006):353-62.

36. ADA Laboratory Evaluation: Bisphenol A Released from Resin-Based Dental Sealants. Volume 10 issue 2; 2015.

37. Cheifetz AT, Osganian SK, Allred EN, Needleman HL. Prevalence of bruxism and associated correlates in children as reported by parents. *J Dent Child* 72, no.2 (2005): 67-73.

38. Sheldon SH. The parasomnias. In: Sheldon SH, Ferber R, Kryger MH, editors. Principles and practice of pediatric sleep medicine. *Elsevier Saunders*; 2005; 305–15.

39. Sari S, Sonmez H. The relationship between occlusal factors and bruxism in permanent and mixed dentition in Turkish children. *J Clin Pediatr Dent* 23, no.3 (2001):191-4.

40. Souto-Souza D, Mourão PS, Barroso HH, Douglas-de-Oliveira DW, Ramos-Jorge ML, Falci SGM, Galvão EL. Is there an association between attention deficit hyperactivity disorder in children and adolescents and the occurrence of bruxism? A systematic review and meta-analysis. *Sleep Med Rev.* 53, (2020): 101330

41. Flores MT, Al Sane M, Andersson L. Information to the public, patients and emergency services on traumatic dental injuries. In: Andreasen JO, Andreasen FM, Andersson L, editors. Textbook and color atlas of traumatic injuries to the teeth. Oxford: Wiley Blackwell, 2019; p. 992–1008.

42. Adnan S, Lone MM, Khan FR, Hussain SM, Nagi SE. Which is the most recommended medium for the storage and transport of avulsed teeth? A systematic review. *Dent Traumatol* 34 (2008): 59–70.

43. Bicak D. A Current Approach to Halitosis and Oral Malodor – A Mini Review. *The Open Dentistry Journal* 12 (2018) 322–330.

44. Kleinberg I, Wolff MS, Codipilly DM. Role of saliva in oral dryness, oral feel, and oral malodor. *Int. Dent. J.* 53, no.3 (2002) 236–240

45. Knapik JJ, Hoedebecke BL, Rogers GG, Sharp MA, Marshall SW. Effectiveness of Mouthguards for the Prevention of Orofacial Injuries and Concussions in Sports: Systematic Review and Meta-Analysis. *Sports Med.* 49, no.8 (2019): 1217-1232.

46. Femanio F, Lanz A, Buonaiuto A, et al. Guidelines for diagnosis and management of aphthous stomatitis. *Pediatr Infect Dis J. 26,* no.8 (2007):728–732.

47   Favia G, Limongelli L, Tempesta A, Maiorano E, Capodiferro S. Oral lesions as first clinical manifestations of Crohn's disease in pediatric patients: a report on 8 cases. *Eur J Paediatr Dent.* 21, no.1 (2020): 66-69.

48   Mochida, Y "Amelogenesis Imperfecta." NORD (National Organization for Rare Disorders), Accessed August 2023. https://rarediseases.org/rare-diseases/amelogenesis-imperfecta/

49   Stanley M. Pathology and epidemiology of HPV infection in females. *Gynecol Oncol* 117, no.2 (2010):S5-10.

50   Rivera C. Essentials of oral cancer. *Int J Clin Exp Pathol* 8 (2015):11884–94.

51   Wodi AP, Murthy N, McNally V, Cineas S, Ault K. Advisory Committee on Immunization Practices Recommended Immunization Schedule for Children and Adolescents Aged 18 Years or Younger — United States, 2023. MMWR Morb Mortal Wkly Rep 2023;72:137–140.

52   Mariotti A, Mawhinney MG. Endocrinology of sex steroid hormones and cell dynamics in the periodontium. *Periodontol* 61, no.1 (2000): 69-88.

53   Southard TE. Third molars and incisor crowding: when removal is unwarranted. J Am Dent Assoc 123, no.8 (1992):75-9.

54   AR Schroder, M Dehghan, TB Newman JP Bentley. Association of Opioid Prescriptions From Dental Clinicians for US Adolescents and Young Adults With Subsequent Opioid Use and Abuse. *Mama Intern Med* 179 vol.2 (2019): 145-152.

55   U.S. Department of Health and Human Services. The Health Consequences of Smoking—50 Years of Progress: A Report of the Surgeon General. Atlanta: U.S. Department of Health and Human Services, Centers for Disease Control and Prevention, National Center for Chronic Disease Prevention and Health Promotion, Office on Smoking and Health, 2014

56   Dietrich T, Walter C, Oluwagbemigun K, Bergmann M, Pischon T, Pischon N, Boeing H. Smoking, Smoking Cessation, and Risk of Tooth Loss: The EPIC-Potsdam Study. *J Dent Res* 94, no.10 (2015):1369-75.

57   U.S. Department of Health and Human Services, Electronic Cigarettes What's the bottom line? Center for Disease Control. September 2023. https://www.cdc.gov/tobacco/basic_information/e-cigarettes/pdfs/Electronic-Cigarettes-Infographic-508.pdf

58   Soneji S, Barrington-Trimis JL, Wills TA, et al. Association between initial use of e-cigarettes and subsequent cigarette smoking among adolescents and young adults: A systematic review and meta-analysis. *JAMA Pediatr* 171, no.8 (2017):788-97.

59   Choi H, Schmidbauer N, Spengler J, Bornehag C. Sources of propylene glycol and glycol ethers in air at home. *Int J Environ Res Public Health* 7, no.12 (2010): 4213-37.

60   U.S. Department of Health and Human Services. The Health Consequences of Smoking – 50 Years of Progress: A Report of the Surgeon General. Rockville, Md.: U.S. Department of Health and Human Services, Centers for Disease Control and Prevention, National Center of Chronic Disease Prevention and Health Promotion, Office on Smoking and Health; 2014.

61   U.S. Department of Health and Human Services. Preventing Tobacco Use Among Youth and Young Adults: A Report of the Surgeon General. Atlanta, Ga.: U.S. Department of Health and Human Services, Centers for Disease Control and Prevention, Office on Smoking and Health; 2012.

62 Fiore MC, Bailey WC, Cohen SJ, et al: Treating tobacco use and dependence. Clinical practice guideline, Rockville, MD, June 2000, US Department of Health and Human Services, Public Health Service.

63 Kukral L, Cruz GD, Dalmas J. Threats to teens' oral health. US Army Center for Health Promotion and Preventive Medicine, Readiness Thru Health 2007: 1-2.

64 Firoozmand LM, Paschotto DR, Almeida JD. Oral piercing complications among teenage students. *Oral Health Prev Dent* 7, no.1 (2009): 77-81.

65 Garcia-Pola MJ, Garcia-Martin JM, Varela-Centelles P, et al. Oral and facial piercing: associated complications and clinical repercussion. *Quintessence Int* 39, no.1 (2008): 51-9.

66 Holbrook J, Minocha J, Laumann A. Body piercing: complications and prevention of health risks. *Am J Clin Dermatol* 13, no.1 (2012): 1-17.

67 Nilsson IM. Reliability, validity, incidence, and impact of temporomandibular pain disorders in adolescents. *Swed Dent J Suppl* 183 (2007): 7-86.

68 Scrivani SJ, Khawaja SN, Bavia PF. Nonsurgical management of pediatric temporomandibular joint dysfunction. *Oral Maxillofac Surg Clin North Am* 30, no.1 (2018): 35-45.

69 List T, Axelsson S, Leijon G. Pharmacologic interventions in the treatment of temporomandibular disorders, atypical facial pain, and burning mouth syndrome. A qualitative systematic review. *J Orofac Pain* 17, no.4 (2003): 301-10.

70 Okeson JP. Temporomandibular joint pains. In Bell's Oral and Facial Pain, 7th edition. Chicago, Ill.: Quintessence Publishing; 2014:327-69.

71 Profitt WR, Fields Jr HW, Server DM. *Contemporary Orthodontics.* 5th ed. Mosby, 2013.

72 American Academy of Dermatology. "Nickel Allergy: How to avoid exposure and reduce symptoms." Accessed December 3, 2023. www.aad.org/public/diseases/eczema/insider/nickel-allergy

73 Tufekci E, Dixon JS, Gunsolley JC, Lindauer SJ. Prevalence of white spot lesions during orthodontic treatment with fixed appliances. *Angle Orthod* 81, (2011):206-10

74 The Heritability of Malocclusion: Part 2. The Influence of Genetics in Malocclusion P.A. Mossey (British Orthodontic Society, 1999).

75 Markovic, M. At the crossroads of orofacial genetics, *European Journal of Orthodontics* 14 no.6 (1992): 469–481.

76 Hsu J, Avila PC, Kern RC, Hayes MC, Schleimer RP, Pinto JM. Genetics of Chronic Rhinosinusitis: State of the Field and Directions Forward. *J Allergy Clin Immunol* 131, no.4 (2013): 977-993

77 Mehta V, Singh RK. Congenitally missing primary and permanent maxillary lateral incisors. *BMJ Case Rep*. Oct 7 (2016) doi: 10.1136/bcr-2016-216779.

78 Polder BJ, Van't Hof MA, Van der Linden FP, Kuijpers-Jagtman AM. A meta-analysis of the prevalence of dental agenesis of permanent teeth. *Community Dent Oral Epidemiol* 32, no.3 (2004): 217-26.

79 Lovgren ML, Dahl O, Urbie P, Ransjo M, Westerlund. Prevalence of impacted maxillary canines – an epidemiological study systematically implemented interceptive treatment. *European Journal of Orthodontics* 41, no.5 (2019): 454-459.

80 Aktan, A.M., Kara, S., Akgunlu, F. and Malkoc, S. The incidence of canine transmigration and tooth impaction in a Turkish subpopulation. *European Journal of Orthodontics* 32, no.5 (2010): 575-581.

81 Brook, A. H. Dental anomalies of number, form, and size: their prevalence in British schoolchildren, *Journal Int Association of Dentistry in Children* 5, no.2 (1974): 37–53.

82 Davis, P. J. Hypodontia and hyperdontia of permanent teeth in Hong Kong schoolchildren, *Community Dentistry and Oral Epidemiology* 15, no.4 (1987): 218–220.

83 Loos, Bruno G, and Thomas E Van Dyke. "The role of inflammation and genetics in periodontal disease." *Periodontology 2000* 83, no.1 (2020): 26-39.

84 Shaddox LM, Morford LA, Nibali L. Periodontal health and disease: The contribution of genetics. *Periodontol* 85, no.1 (2021):161-181.

85 Vieira AR. Genetics and Caries: prospects. *Braz Oral Res.* 26, no.1 (2012): 7-9.

86 Centers for Disease Control and Prevention (CDC). National Center for Health Statistics (NCHS). National Health and Nutrition Examination Survey Data. Hyattsville, MD: U.S. Department of Health and Human Services, Centers for Disease Control and Prevention, [2014]

87 Oh TJ, Eber R, Wang HL. Periodontal diseases in the child and adolescent. *Journal of Clinical Periodontology* 29, no.5 (2002): 400-10.

88 Brown, LJ, Löe H. Prevalence, extent, severity and progression of periodontal disease. *Periodontology 2000* 2, no.1 (1993): 57-71.

89 Ciancio SG, Medications' impact on oral health. *The Journal of the American Dental Association* 135, no.10 (2004):1440-1448.

90 Bharti V, Bansal C. Drug-induced gingival overgrowth: The nemesis of gingiva unraveled. *J Indian Soc Periodontol.* 17, no.2 (2013): 182-187.

91 Zucchelli, Giovanni, and Ilham Mounssif. Periodontal plastic surgery. *Periodontology 2000* 68, no.1 (2015): 333-68

92 King, Shalinie et al. Oral health and cardiometabolic disease: understanding the relationship. *Internal medicine journal* 52, no.2 (2022): 198-205.

93 American Academy of Sleep Medicine. International Classification of Sleep Disorders, 3rd ed. Darien, Ill.: American Academy of Sleep Medicine; 2014:63-8.

94 American Academy of Sleep Medicine. Rising prevalence of sleep apnea in U.S. threatens public health. 2014. Available at: https://aasm.org/rising-prevalence-of-sleep-apnea-in-u-s-threatens-public-health/ – :~:text=DARIEN, IL – Sept.,National Healthy Sleep Awareness Project. Accessed June 24, 2021.

95 Stark TR, Pozo-Alonso M, Daniels R, Camacho M. Pediatric considerations for dental sleep medicine. *Sleep Med Clin* 13, no.8 (2018):531-48.

INDEX

A

anticipatory guidance 16

B

bacteria 16, 20, 27, 44, 151, 154, 162
bad breath (halitosis) 74, 75
bite issues

    anterior crossbite 76
    crowding 78, 105
    malocclusions 110
    open-bite 43, 78, 108, 134, 144
    overbite 108, 120, 143
    overjet 79, 108
    posterior crossbite 76, 112
    underbite 109, 131, 135, 137, 143

bottle 20, 26
breastfeeding 25, 26
brushing 59, 84, 93, 129

    starting 19
    technique 21, 24, 37
    toothbrush 38

C

cavities 20, 27, 44, 64, 93, 148
cleft lip and palate 12

D

dental visits 34, 62

    first visit 16
    rehearsal visit 40

diet 6, 20, 26, 42, 125

F

fear (phobia) 39
flossing 25, 37, 59, 74, 84, 139
fluoride 22, 23, 24, 25, 62, 93, 129
frenum 85, 158, 169

G

gastroesophageal reflux disease (GERD) 74, 87
genetics 142, 148
gingiva

    bumps 19
    pigmentation 157

gingivitis 74, 84, 94, 151
grinding 63, 64, 102, 143

H

HPV (Human Papilloma Virus) 89

I

impaction (stuck tooth)

    canine 146
    ectopic molar 65

infections

    abscess 154
    swelling 27, 44

L

lasers 64

M

mouth breathing 75, 78, 144
mouthguard 83, 84, 126
mouthwashes 39, 62

O

obstructive sleep apnea (OSA) 161

    snoring 78

orthodontic treatment

    aligners (trays) 126
    bite bumps 120
    bite turbos 120
    braces 114, 116, 118, 121
    complications 119, 121, 124, 125, 130
    elastics 122, 123
    expansion 78, 111, 113, 114
    headgear 131
    hygiene considerations 129, 131
    orthognathic surgery 136
    retainers 99, 138, 140
    timing 104

P

periodontitis 12, 101, 148, 152
phase 1 93, 105
phase 2 105, 114
piercings 102
plaque 74, 84, 129, 150, 151, 153

    tartar 151, 153

pregnancy 6, 10, 11

R

recession 88, 102, 155, 156, 158

S

sealants 60, 61, 62
sedation 45, 46
sensitivity 88, 155
shark teeth 53
smoking 101
space

    creating space 105
    diastema 85

space maintainers 37, 82
speech 12, 79
sucking habits 28, 43, 77, 132

T

teeth

    color 33, 56
    formation 9, 22, 33
    layers 27, 56, 94
    number 8, 19, 33, 52, 53, 144
    shape 54, 57, 144
    timing 17, 18, 48, 51, 66
    types 6

teething 15, 91
thrush 29
timing 104
TMJ (temporomandibular joint) 102
tongue-tie 28, 158
tonsils and adenoids 78, 162, 163
toothaches 40, 98
toothpaste 21, 24, 37, 59, 88, 129
trauma

    adult teeth 67, 69
    baby teeth 27, 41

treatment

    fillings and crowns 94
    implants 95
    root canal 94

U

ulcers

    canker sores (aphthous ulcers) 85
    Herpetic Gingivostomatitis 30
    illness related 87
    post-anesthesia lip biting 44

W

whitening (bleaching) 100
wisdom teeth (third molars) 96, 97, 98, 144

X

X-rays 34, 35